ADVANCED CONSULTING IN FAMILY MEDICINE

THE CONSULTATION EXPERTISE MODEL

Edited by

PETER WORRALL
Educator and Founder Member of Leicester Simulated Patient Unit

ADRIAN FRENCH
Family Doctor
Former Course Organiser and Programme Director

and

LES ASHTON
Family Doctor – GP Revalidation Lead, NHS Leicester City
and Former Programme Director

Foreword by

JUSTIN ALLEN
Special Adviser on Quality and Programmes
UK Foundation Programme Office, Cardiff
Honorary Professor of Family Medicine
De Montfort University, Leicester

Radcliffe Publishing
Oxford • New York

Radcliffe Publishing Ltd
18 Marcham Road
Abingdon
Oxon OX14 1AA
United Kingdom

www.radcliffe-oxford.com

Electronic catalogue and worldwide online ordering facility.

British Library Cataloguing in Publication Data

A catalogue record for this book is available from the British Library.

ISBN-13: 978 184619 180 0

Typeset by Pindar NZ, Auckland, New Zealand
Printed and bound by TJI Digital, Padstow, Cornwall, UK

CONTENTS

Foreword   v
About the authors   vii
Acknowledgements   x
List of figures   xii

**1 INTRODUCTION TO THE CONSULTATION
    EXPERTISE MODEL**   1
What is *Advanced Consulting* about?   1
Consultation Expertise Model: context   5
Who is *Advanced Consulting* written for?   6
Why is the Consultation Expertise Model of value?   7
Assumptions   9
Issues arising   14

2 THE CONSULTATION EXPERTISE MODEL   17
The four components of the Model   17
1. What we mean by – consulting skills   20
2. Domains of expertise   33
3. What we mean by – performance levels   60
4. What we mean by – indicative statements   65
Using indicative statements – an illustrative case   67
Advanced consulting – a summary   96

3 FINGERPRINTING   101
The Impression Graph   101
Making a fingerprint   105
Common marking problems   110
Giving feedback using the Consultation Expertise Model   113

Feedback example: the case of Mrs Judith Anderson   116
Feedback – using a case narrative   125

4   USES OF THE MODEL   129
Introducing the Consultation Expertise Model to colleagues   129
Using the Consultation Expertise Model for appraisal and revalidation   132
Use by a practising family doctor – feedback from a colleague using the
      Consultation Expertise Model for self-reflection   133
Use by a family doctor trainer   138
Use with a family doctor trainer group   140

**5   ADVANCED CONSULTING AND THE MODEL:
KEY CONCEPTS   144**
Key concepts in relation to 'consulting skills'   144
Key concepts in relation to the Impression Graph   150
Key concepts in relation to expertise training   154

**6   PRACTICAL APPROACHES TO DEVELOPING ADVANCED
CONSULTING EXPERTISE   163**
Establishing a mindset and direction of travel   163
Designing an expertise teaching programme: preliminary thoughts   170

Appendix 1: The Consultation Expertise Model: the developmental journey   174
Appendix 2: The question of validity and reliability   192
Appendix 3: The use of simulated patients   196
Appendix 4: Fingerprint Pack   200

Index   217

FOREWORD

One of the most valued memories of my long career as a general practice educator is that of working with the team of simulated patients in the postgraduate general practice department at Leicester, in producing a consulting skills assessment method for general practice vocational training. During this process these simulators would consult as patients with a range of consulters, ranging from medical students to family doctor directors. During discussions after a working session, simulators would often say that they, as patients, could easily distinguish when they were consulting with a competent newly qualified family doctor and a new trainee, but what was more surprising was that they could also easily distinguish between a newly qualified family doctor and a trainer, even when of comparable age. This started a discussion within the team – how did they know? What was different? The result is in your hands.

Expertise in consulting is key to the provision of high-quality patient care in family medicine. In these days of rapid advances in bio-technical ways of delivering healthcare, the humanistic skills of the family doctor are needed more than ever. How can we ensure that these skills are maintained and developed throughout medical education, in the continuum from undergraduate education to specialty training and continuing professional development?

The conceptual framework of a continuum of skilled behaviour from the competent to proficient to expert was not developed for application in the general practice consulting setting but clearly is needed. In some family doctors' hands consulting may have become a high art. How do practitioners move themselves towards becoming an expert consulter? A further factor is that of the complexity of general practice itself and the multitude of tasks a family doctor has to undertake in each consultation. It is clear from this book that expert consulting is similarly complex. The authors have identified and described eight domains of consulting activity. Within each of these they have gone on to describe three levels of consulting expertise through indicative statements. They have recognised that in consulting with patients individual doctors may vary in their level of expertise from domain to domain, and external factors may bring about variability day to day.

The Model can be applied at different levels. Those in specialty training will find it useful in becoming competent in consulting. Every newly qualified family doctor will wish to build on the work they did with their trainer to continue to improve their consulting skills. Using this Model individual family doctors can identify their own pattern of expertise, using the eight domains. Through a process of reflection and feedback they are enabled to move their consulting skills to higher levels.

Until now there has been little written about advanced consulting skills and there have been few practical models to help this essential process of lifelong learning. This book provides an excellent, clear practical guide for all those doctors interested in becoming better at consulting with patients. It is essential reading for family doctor educators.

Professor Justin Allen
Special Adviser on Quality and Programmes
UK Foundation Programme Office, Cardiff
Honorary Professor of Family Medicine
De Montfort University, Leicester
November 2008

ABOUT THE AUTHORS

The Consultation Expertise Model has been collectively constructed by:

Les Ashton

Les Ashton has been a family doctor for nearly 20 years and works in an inner-city Leicester practice dealing solely with primary care for asylum seekers. He has been a programme director and Balint group facilitator for the East Midlands Healthcare Workforce Deanery. His main areas of interests are primary care mental health and consultation skills. He is a member of the RCGP mental health task group and also the Curriculum and Development Lead for PRIMHE, a primary care mental health and education charity. He is a member of the RCGP Curriculum Development Steering Group.

Adrian French

Consideration for patients' realities did not figure prominently in Adrian's early training. It was when, in a northern city, his trainer gave him a lexicon of the local patois that his interests in the subtler skills of consulting really took off. Over the past 25 years he has refined this ability in a variety of socially and ethnically diverse practices and as a course organiser/programme director. He has been part of a team of people refining their use of patient simulation for training and assessment at local and national level. Recently, he has become an enthusiast for composting, a slow and sometimes mysterious process which he considers a useful metaphor for the development of consulting expertise.

Sarah Greening

Sarah is a part-time family doctor in Northampton town centre. Her clinical interests include women's health, mental health and palliative medicine. She is a family doctor trainer – a role that maintains her motivation for the job and also keeps her on her toes. In addition, she is the GP appraisal lead for Northamptonshire PCT – a challenging role but one that allows her to channel her interests in innovation and support of colleagues. Consultation skills are pivotal to all of her roles, including family life, where planning and negotiation are vital components particularly with her two children.

Simon Gregory

Simon Gregory has been a family doctor in inner-city Northampton for 13 years. Having gone to the area to get married, he has been there ever since. His particular clinical interests include respiratory medicine, mental health and women's health. He is GP postgraduate dean for the East Midlands, a role he thrives on but not one which helps his carbon footprint. He is also editor in chief of *General Practice Update*, an elected member of the RCGP council and a vice-chair of COGPED. With two teenage daughters the grey hairs have started to sprout, so when he can he escapes into his 'cave' to turn wood.

Bevis Heap

Bevis sees himself as a 'jobbing' family doctor with, as his recent appraiser said, 'fingers in lots of pies'. He has been in practice for 22 years and a trainer for much of that. He has an interest in mental health and was a hospital practitioner in psychiatry for some years. Being a trainer and a tutor on new trainers' courses makes consultation skills a very important part of his working life. Outside work he relaxes by playing trains, among other things.

Nick Leach

After six years as an inner-London family doctor, where he undertook Balint training at the Tavistock Institute, Nick emigrated to rural Leicestershire, where he has practised for the last 29 years. A large population of travellers local to his practice has led him to set up an enhanced service designed to reduce their very high levels of morbidity. He has been a family doctor trainer for the last 26 years and this experience has taught him the importance of consultation expertise as central to effective primary care. He has also been an appraiser, is currently chairman of his GP locality forum and is appointed to the chair of the Leicestershire RCGP faculty.

Megan Murray

After studying Mandarin, Megan spent time as a teacher in the hinterland of China. This spurred her interest in language usage and in the UK she has taught international students at the University of Leicester and spent many a long hour poring over scripts and proof-reading for colleagues. Megan is also a simulated patient and joined the project when the Model's indicative statements were under scrutiny.

Paul Platts

Paul qualified as a doctor in 1975 and followed in his grandfather and father's footsteps, entering family medicine in a suburban area with significant elements of deprivation. He became a trainer after four years and was a course organiser for just under 20 years. His suburban practice had a higher than average consultation rate which started his interest in developing his consulting skills further. This led to an interest in exploring the characteristics of an expert consultation.

Tim Smith

Tim has been a principal in family medicine in a Leicestershire market town for 28 years and a family doctor trainer for nearly as long. A few years ago, in order to stave off something or other, he took up windsurfing. As with higher-order consulting it raised the question of how to recognise an expert. It's obvious when you watch one but to try and break the skills down and teach them is another matter. It is that which attracted him to the project, along with the hope that some of the consulting skills identified might stick to him – with the added bonus of not getting wet.

Peter Worrall

Peter taught in schools for over 30 years, much of that time as a principal of schools with parallel community programmes. While working in educational management as an associate lecturer with the Open University he became involved with the development of simulated patients for the assessment of consultation skills. He started and ran the Leicester Simulated Patient Unit for some years. This, together with his involvement as a non-clinical VTS course organiser, led to a deeper involvement in medical education. Imprinted from his former practice is the belief that high learning expectations are essential for high achievement, hence his curiosity about higher-order consulting skills.

ACKNOWLEDGEMENTS

The Consultation Expertise Model emerged at Leicester VTS during a period when dialogue about the quality of family doctor postgraduate training was an engrossing weekly preoccupation. Corridor conversations led to exploration of varied group work approaches, away days and design of new resources. The commitment to improve the quality of training was high on the agenda. It was in this atmosphere that questions about the nature of higher-order family doctor consulting arose.

This spirit of enquiry was endorsed and encouraged by successive directors of postgraduate GP education, David Sowden and Justin Allen. It was David who took the farsighted decision to kick-start this enquiry and thereafter Justin whose vision provided firm support, both creatively and practically, over many years. It is to Justin that we owe the suggestion to present the Model in circular format. We would like to thank them both for the enthusiastic communication of their vision, availability for advice and unending support.

Many elements of the Model evolved from the development of patient simulations in various health centres around the county. While this work was innovative and exciting, it often took place in the evening after surgery, enlivened by engagement with the 'patients'. We would like to thank all the simulators, the practices and their staff who participated in and played host to our activities.

We are grateful for the scrutiny provided at a crucial time in the Model's development by the Family Medicine Faculty of the RC University of Leuven, Belgium, and the participants from many parts of Europe who attended workshops at WONCA meetings.

Over the years many family doctor specialist registrars have helped us make significant modifications to our thinking about the concepts underlying the Model and the uses it could or should be put to. We hope they have learned as much from us as we have from them.

Chris Cooper-Hayes of C3 Creative has played visual nurse to the project over many years. His patience in translating our scribbles into something that others might understand has been invaluable.

The following family doctors and simulator colleagues have at various times helped the project along its wayward path. Without their encouragement and assistance the project would have withered years ago. Heena Bharkada, Frank Callow, Gareth Chidlow, Alistair Craig, Mike Drucquer, Julie Duke, Nick Gravestock, Michele Gutteridge, Tim Hammond, Anna Hiley, Bridget Kielty, Tim Jennings, David Kerbel, Rhona Knight, John Middleton, Tim Norfolk, Carolyn Oldershaw, Andy Reeves, David Shepherd, Tanya Sperry, Pete Wells, Marcus Wilde, Martin Williams and Brenda Worrall.

LIST OF FIGURES

1.01	The Consultation Expertise Model	xvi
1.02a, 1.02b	Case fingerprints: what they might look like	4
1.03	Mind map of factors affecting the consultation	10
1.04	Adapted Miller Triangle	13
2.01	Consulting skills core	17
2.02	Circle with eight domains	18
2.03	Circle with three performance levels	19
2.04	Indicative statements for Communication domain	19
2.05	Consulting skills – essential skills at the core of the Model	20
2.06	Consulting skills showing idea of extended growth of key skills	22
2.07	Critical application of medical knowledge and skills – features of skill development	22
2.08	Complex clinical problem framing and solving skills	24
2.09	Extended interpersonal skills	27
2.10	The computer – symbol of the external world	30
2.11	The most important consulting skills variable	31
2.12	Consulting skills developing in parallel with clinical performance	32
2.13	Communication – domain segment	33
2.14	Recognising Patterns – domain segment	36
2.15	Medical Competence – domain segment	39
2.16	Respecting Patients – domain segment	42
2.17	Dealing with Uncertainty – domain segment	45
2.18	Use of Resources – domain segment	49
2.19	Focus – domain segment	53
2.20	Synthesising Skills – domain segment	57
2.21	Performance staging posts	64
2.22	The Model so far – consulting skills + domains + performance levels	65

2.23   Using indicative statements to determine expertise levels is akin
        to pond dipping   69
2.24   Communication – domain with indicative statements +
        marking key   72
2.25   Communication – fingerprint markings   75
2.26   Recognising Patterns – domain with indicative statements +
        marking key   76
2.27   Recognising Patterns – fingerprint markings   77
2.28   Medical Competence – domain with indicative statements +
        marking key   79
2.29   Medical Competence – fingerprint markings   81
2.30   Respecting Patients – domain with indicative statements +
        marking key   82
2.31   Respecting Patients – fingerprint markings   84
2.32   Dealing with Uncertainty – domain with indicative statements +
        marking key   85
2.33   Dealing with Uncertainty – fingerprint markings   87
2.34   Use of Resources – domain with indicative statements +
        marking key   88
2.35   Use of Resources – fingerprint markings   90
2.36   Focus – domain with indicative statements + marking key   91
2.37   Focus – fingerprint markings   93
2.38   Synthesising Skills with indicative statements + marking key   94
2.39   Synthesising Skills – fingerprint markings   95
3.01   The Impression Graph   102
3.02   Impression Graph capture of expertise for two doctors
        consulting with the same patient simulation   104
3.03   Marked Impression Graph alongside a fingerprint of the
        same case   109
3.04   Experienced doctor – typical six fingerprints with case related
        challenge   111
3.05   Judith Anderson: experienced family doctor specialist
        registrar – fingerprint and Impression Graph   119
3.06   Judith Anderson: experienced family doctor – fingerprint and
        Impression Graph   124
4.01   Marked fingerprint and Impression Graph   136
5.01   Example of an extended interpersonal skill – cues and clues   147
5.02   Example of an extended interpersonal skill – questioning   148
5.03   Example of an extended skilled clinical behaviour – negotiation   149

5.04	Example of an interpersonal skills overview	150
6.01	Relationship of the 'concepts' to the Impression Graph	169
6.02	Elements in a teaching programme	172
A.1	The linear model	175
A.2	Illustration of case treatment progression	175
A.3	Fingerprints showing variation at four experience levels	177
A.4	Six fingerprints showing variation according to case challenge	179
A.5	Judith Anderson – comparison fingerprints	180
A.6	Impression Graph	182

NOTE TO UK READERS

To reflect the international readership the terms 'family doctor' and 'family practice' are used rather than the UK-specific 'GP' and 'general practice'.

Consultation Expertise Model

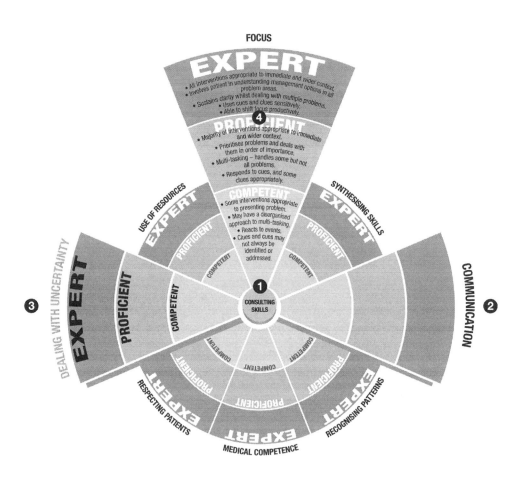

FOCUS

EXPERT
- All interventions appropriate to immediate and wider context.
- Involves patient in understanding management options in all problem areas.
- Sustains clarity whilst dealing with multiple problems.
- Uses cues and clues sensitively.
- Able to shift focus productively.

④

PROFICIENT
- Majority of interventions appropriate to immediate and wider context.
- Prioritises problems and deals with them in order of importance.
- Multi-tasking – handles some but not all problems.
- Responds to cues, and some clues appropriately.

COMPETENT
- Some interventions appropriate to presenting problem.
- May have a disorganised approach to multi-tasking.
- Reacts to events.
- Clues and cues may not always be identified or addressed.

USE OF RESOURCES · EXPERT · PROFICIENT · COMPETENT

SYNTHESISING SKILLS · EXPERT · PROFICIENT · COMPETENT

① CONSULTING SKILLS

③ DEALING WITH UNCERTAINTY · EXPERT · PROFICIENT · COMPETENT

② COMMUNICATION

COMPETENT · PROFICIENT · EXPERT · RECOGNISING PATTERNS

RESPECTING PATIENTS · EXPERT · PROFICIENT · COMPETENT

MEDICAL COMPETENCE

The four components

❶	**❷**	**❸**	**❹**
Consulting Skills	**Domains**	**Performance Levels**	**Indicative Statements**
Medical Knowledge and Skills	Communication	Competent	For each
Problem Framing and Solving	Recognising Patterns	Proficient	performance level
Interpersonal Skills	Medical Competence	Expert	of each domain
	Respecting Patients		
	Dealing with Uncertainty		
	Use of Resources		
	Focus		
	Synthesising skills		

Figure 1.01 The Consultation Expertise Model

1 INTRODUCTION TO THE CONSULTATION EXPERTISE MODEL

WHAT IS *ADVANCED CONSULTING* ABOUT?

> 'Fulfilment and excellence should be the goals, and deserve to be the destiny, of anyone embarking on a Vocational Training Apprenticeship . . . The trouble is, "fulfilment" appears to be a will-o'-the-wisp; and despite our chasing it with a net made of objectives and checklists, "excellence" tantalisingly evades capture, no matter how fine the mesh.'[1]

Consulting: it's what family doctors do every day, week in week out until it's taken for granted. By some that is. For experienced doctors it appears easy: sit down, glance at the screen and, 'Hello, how are you?' Just as the skilled musician takes up an instrument, looks at the score and plays a perfect series of notes to make music that is personally idiosyncratic and yet moves others. Ask these experts to describe what they are doing and the answer may be something akin to, 'I don't know. I just do it' – what Daniel Barenboim in the 2006 BBC Reith Lectures called 'conscious naivety'. This is fine for reassured patients or music lovers but it is very frustrating for teachers. They like to know what's going on and want answers to questions such as:

- What exactly do experienced family doctors do?
- What distinguishes expert family doctors from their colleagues?

It shouldn't be such a mystery!

> 'A diverse group of case studies illustrates the grounding of skill in physical practice – the hand habits of striking a piano key or using a knife; the written recipes used to guide the neophyte cook; the use of imperfect scientific instruments like the first telescopes or puzzling instruments like the anatomist's scalpel; . . . Developing skill in all these domains is arduous, but it is not mysterious.'[2]

It's about the way experienced doctors consult

We were prompted to explore these questions by people working as simulated patients in specialist training for family medicine. They studied, in great detail, recordings of patients made in daily surgeries in order to develop simulations. The simulation is subsequently used with doctors in training as well as by experienced practitioners.[3] As the simulator recreates the same patient to each of these doctors, perhaps inevitably they make comparisons. They tell of being aware of the cogs going round in the heads of family doctor trainees, with cog rotation punctuated by pauses that resonate with messages such as, 'What do I ask next?' By contrast they describe consultations with more experienced doctors as seamless, easy, relaxed or sometimes even puzzlingly unpredictable. Hence the question: 'What distinguishes the consulting of experienced family doctors from their newly qualified colleagues?' At the time there appeared to be no easily available answer that could be used by medical educators. This book provides an answer.

Advanced Consulting presents a schematic representation of what expert family doctors actually do. It avoids tantalising value judgement such as 'excellence', but describes expert behaviours in terms that can be observed day to day. The Consultation Expertise Model, hereafter referred to as the Model, illustrates in practical terms how the quality of consulting performance may develop over the years, given time for reflection and a commitment to learn from experience.

It is not surprising that one question necessarily leads on to another. In most fields of professional endeavour there is a clear understanding of what constitutes best practice, together with appropriately staged training for those practitioners who aspire to reach higher levels of practice. This is exemplified in many secondary care specialisms. However, while family doctors may extend their expertise into areas of special interest or needs – minor surgery, sexual health or asylum seekers, for example – there is no universal expertise-related training available post certification or accreditation. Given the above, the Model seeks to provide a detailed picture of *what* constitutes advanced consulting behaviour, i.e. best practice. Furthermore, it seeks to establish *how* changes in behaviour can be identified and evaluated and *how* family doctors can be helped to acquire these higher levels of expertise.

As the ideas embedded in the Model came together it became possible to express them graphically in a circular format as can be seen in Figure 1.02. This allows the Model to be used as a tool to 'map' consultations. Consultation mapping is a familiar technique introduced by Pendleton *et al.*[4] and elaborated by Tate.[5] The circular 'map' generated using the Model is called a fingerprint.

It's about capturing excellence in the consultation through 'fingerprinting'

A fingerprint is a form of consultation capture directly related to the Model that diagrammatises behaviour observed at different performance levels – always case-specific. Fingerprints made according to the criteria of the Model provide evidence on which to base discussion of what happened, what might have happened and, had behaviour been different, prompt thinking about future intentions that can be included in a learning plan.

Please note – a consultation map plots how events during the consultation pass through predetermined domains (e.g. establishing reasons for attendance) over a period of time whereas a fingerprint presents a holistic record of skills demonstrated in the consultation as a whole.

Using paperwork in the Fingerprint Pack provided in Appendix 4, post-fingerprint discussions contribute to a continuing professional development (CPD) process that can be included in appraisal or revalidation folders. The facility to fingerprint consultations, as will be explained later, enables expertise development to be identified and evaluated. Fingerprints can be expressed in two different ways as shown in Figure 1.02.

It's about how consulting expertise may be developed

Finding a way to identify what expert family doctors do turns out to be the easy part. Having obtained a picture of advanced consulting, the question of how to achieve the higher performance levels identified must inevitably follow. There is little point in dangling an enticing picture of what experts do in front of family doctors early in their careers when they are still consolidating and extending their range of experience. That would be frustrating and counterproductive for all concerned. Indeed the new doctor will have been in daily contact with expert behaviour by their trainer and mentor but will be unable to copy it because the gap between competent and expert behaviour is incomprehensible to them without an aid to analysis. Experts make it look easy. How can you copy a relaxed and knowing manner that has taken years of experience to achieve?

Ways to benefit from experience will be suggested later in the book. The Model itself incorporates detailed next-stage suggestions which, in conjunction with the fingerprinting process, can provide further direction and insight. In addition, three key approaches central to expert behaviour and usable for self-development or as taught workshops will be outlined as routes to an extended consultation expertise repertoire.

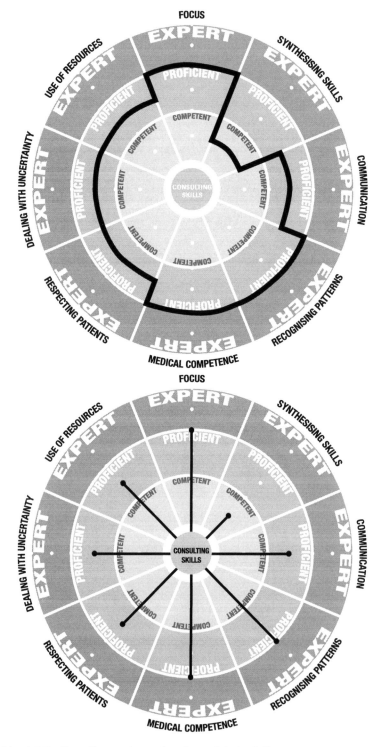

Figures 1.02a, 1.02b Case fingerprints: what they might look like

> *Advanced Consulting* is about the development and growth of existing skills which have been learned by all family doctors by the time of certification.

At this point you may be thinking 'Oh no, not something else to worry about'. However, the Model should be regarded not as another added pressure, but as a new way of looking at how existing skills are being used. Indeed, for many practitioners who have used it, it has evoked a revelation and provided the language for a reaction of, 'Oh, that's what I've been doing, is it?'

Advanced Consulting is written in handbook form for easy access and use. The Model and fingerprint process is explained stage by stage so that fingerprints can be made at home for personal reflection, for mutual exchange or within a practice organisation for dialogue between colleagues. Whichever approach is chosen, the resulting fingerprint can be used as evidence of professional development for the doctor who did the consultation.

In addition, the Model provides, maybe even provokes, a language and a vision of higher-order family doctor consulting for debate and celebration of professional skill. Another possible bonus is the prospect of acquiring internal staging posts to stimulate the intrinsic reward that can come from growth of expertise. In Roger Neighbour's terms, as quoted at the beginning of this introduction, we have found this a fulfilling experience.

Finally, *Advanced Consulting* may be regarded as an exploration of expert doctoring *for its own sake*.

CONSULTATION EXPERTISE MODEL: CONTEXT

It is important to emphasise just how influential local factors have been in sustaining interest in this question of expertise. Three local context factors stand out. First, most of those involved have become familiar over the years with a nationally known consulting skill development framework devised and used locally for undergraduate training: the Leicester Assessment Package (LAP).[6] LAP provides the basis for systematic training and assessment in the University of Leicester Medical School and is used by family doctor trainers with medical students. Patient simulators are also familiar with the methodology as they participate as patients in student action learning workshops.

Second, members of the group have been integrally involved in the development of patient simulations based on recordings of actual patients in real family doctor situations, not on written scenarios. As a consequence, the project group has had access to experienced simulators from the Leicester Simulated Patient Unit[7] who are accustomed to looking at videotapes of experienced doctor consultations. Being able to compare different doctors consulting with the same simulated patient is a unique resource used frequently by the project group.

Third, some of the work on the competencies necessary for the selection and future training of family doctors involved local medical educators and simulators.[8,9] This involvement influenced our thinking to ensure that the Model developed in a way that was consistent with curriculum development and professional training.

As a consequence of these three factors, eight family doctors concerned with education and training sustained a voluntary interest in the project over seven years with modest development funds to assist their enquiry.

It is necessary to emphasise the Model's educational provenance. Although improved health outcomes have been implicit in all aspects of group thinking, the driving force for this project has been educational – to discover insights that will aid the growth of expertise and fulfilment. Furthermore, in retrospect, the manner in which the project has explored the issue can be seen to fit an educational action research model[10,11] more comfortably than conventional medical research.

The book therefore arises out of local contextual influences and is composed of contributions from all members of the project team and valued local colleagues (*see* Appendix 1 for the full story of the Model's development).

WHO IS *ADVANCED CONSULTING* WRITTEN FOR?

Advanced Consulting provides the means to evaluate what is happening in any one or in a series of family doctor consultations. The fingerprinting process provides the means to identify what happens in any one consultation on a performance spectrum with a view to exploring stages of expertise. The overriding purpose of the Model is to encourage interest in the development of high-quality expert level consulting *for its own sake* and, by extension, for continuing professional development (CPD). We will emphasise many times that the Consultation Expertise Model is intended for formative, personal use only. It is not validated for summative assessment. To that end the Model is designed for anyone interested in exploring how they consult.

> The Consultation Expertise Model is for formative, personal use only; it is not validated for assessment.

The project group started out with the intention of identifying what experienced doctors do in order to provide doctors about to finish their training with a picture – a mental map of high-quality consulting against which they could later judge their own performance. This idea became secondary when we discovered how difficult it was for trainee family doctors to appreciate what was happening in an apparently effortless consultation, despite appropriate medical outcomes and patient satisfaction. This made us very cautious about introducing talk of expert consulting before new doctors were ready to look too far ahead. That aside, it was the discovery of the fingerprinting process that shifted the focus of the Model to providing a useful tool for all practising family doctors.

We now consider that the Model can be used by:

- family doctor trainers with trainees whose level of competence, prior to full-time practice, is ready for the challenge of what they might do to improve their performance still further
- family doctor educators with groups of trainees near to certification who will benefit from a longer-term picture of expertise progression
- any practising family doctor who wishes, either alone or with a colleague, to explore how they are consulting
- practising doctors or doctors from more doctor-centred cultures who need or wish to review their consulting skills
- practitioners who want to explore their consulting to provide evidence for appraisal or revalidation folders.

The Consultation Expertise Model has been devised by practitioners for practitioners – it is a doctor-centred model predicated on a patient-centred approach. However, the nature of expertise featured in the following pages may also be of interest to a more academic audience whose interests lie more generally in the process of professional skill development.

WHY IS THE CONSULTATION EXPERTISE MODEL OF VALUE?
It is the purpose of the Model to inform and motivate the growth of expertise.

For family doctors in training
So intensive is the training process prior to certification that there is little room in trainees' heads for a model that projects them beyond their immediate concerns. Nevertheless, when trainees are sufficiently confident in their consulting ability (as many who pass the required assessments prior to the end of training are) the Model can be used by trainers when tutoring, to extend expertise using discrete aspects of the Model; for example, one component of the Model considers the problem of dealing with uncertainty at different performance levels.

> The Consultation Expertise Model can provide, or illuminate, a progressive pathway to high-quality consulting performance for newly certified family doctors.

For experienced practitioners

Doctors do not often see each other consult; unless there is a chaperone, student or registrar present, the consultation is a confidential private act between patient and doctor. Even if there is the will, there are a range of practical problems in the way of colleague observation: sufficient surgery time to double-up, personality issues, resistance or reticence, to mention just four. Though exposure to colleagues may be initially risky, the Consultation Expertise Model does provide an opportunity to break out of this lonely mould. For someone who has never recorded a consultation before it is easy enough to sort out the practicalities. One needs look no further than the following quotation to find reasons why this may be desirable.

> *'Feedback of one sort or another is essential to all skill acquisition. One cannot improve unless one has ways of judging how good present performance is, and in which direction change must occur.'*[12]

The Model is not constructed with any kind of performance *definition* in mind; it is made for dialogue based on performance description. In an internal dialogue, 'Why did I do that?', 'Am I only competent or was that because of the low case challenge?', 'Wow am I that good?', the Model provides an alternative to personal opinion. It is an inherently safe activity because control is largely in the hands of the user.

Having used the Model privately, the next step is to exchange tapes with a trusted colleague. It is worth emphasising that using the Model correctly as the basis for unpacking what happens in a consultation will avoid the danger of potentially being hurt by unsupported opinion. The Model (as do other models) provides the evidence for a developmental dialogue.

> The intrinsic reward for recognition of improvement in expertise is job satisfaction.

For appraisal and revalidation

Central to the supporting paperwork for the Model is a final page on which doctors record what the outcomes of the dialogue have directed them to do next in order to influence their performance, with the overall aim of improving personal and patient satisfaction. These outcomes can be included in an appraisal or revalidation folder and used as evidence both of performance levels and commitment to CPD.

> For doctors familiar with the Model there is economy of use; both for enjoyable, professional discussion and the provision of evidence for appraisal and revalidation procedures.

ASSUMPTIONS

The Consultation Expertise Model has implications for every family doctor. Just glancing at it must in some ways prompt an internal dialogue, even a challenge, to lived experience in the practice: 'Is that what I do?', 'Why should I do that?', 'They've got that wrong'. We do accept the Model will raise all kinds of questions prior to any decision to use it, so we feel it necessary to share some of the assumptions we've made and as such provide a necessary preparation for the reader to approach the Model at face value.

- A clarification: the title *Advanced Consulting* should be taken as being synonymous with the aspiration to achieve expert-level consultations.
- We take as a given that no doctor can be considered expert unless they have developed insights through acquiring extensive knowledge and understanding of medical conditions together with sufficient creativity to use those insights in the resolution of different patients' problems. This requires several years in practice.
- The assumption that the doctor has a competent level of medical knowledge and skill allows us freedom to concentrate more specifically on the interaction between doctor and patient in the application of that knowledge.
- While concentrating on the confounding variables between doctor and patient, it should not be assumed that the authors are unaware of the many other factors which impact on the quality of the consultation from time to time. Some of these may certainly inhibit attention to expertise development. Figure 1.03 below reflects the wide and varied influences a group of experienced trainers considered to impinge on the way a consultation may be conducted.

In general, consultation models either provide approaches and frameworks to *consult well*: Pendleton,[13] Neighbour,[14] Cambridge-Calgary[15] or to consult in *particular ways*: Helman,[16] McWhinney/Stewart[17,18] or Elwyn.[19] We assume here that most family doctors enter the profession with a professional awareness of these models and a

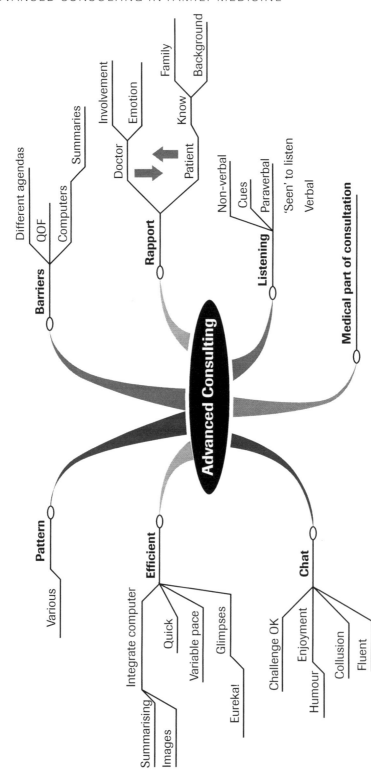

Figure 1.03 Mind map of factors affecting the consultation

consultation style that suits their abilities and value systems. Their consulting style may also have been influenced by the preferences of their trainer(s). We make the assumption, therefore, that the approach taken by new doctors will reflect an amalgam of recommended practice.

- In using the Consultation Expertise Model we assume doctors have been certified medically competent to practise (the Model is not at all useful as a measure of competence in the sense of a doctor being competent to practise). The **competent performance level of the Model relates to a good consultation**.

- As an extension of the above it can also be assumed that the **progression from competent to expert is by addition of insights and applications to existing skills** in a uniquely individual way that results in an extended repertoire of consulting behaviours.

  'Each person brings his own particular history, intellectual commitments and readiness to learn to a particular clinical situation.'[20]

- It can be assumed that some doctors entering the profession will already be working at a proficient level in some domains. It is unlikely, however, unless they are exceptional, that such doctors will reach expert level because **expert level is predicated on extended practice**. By definition, 'recognising patterns', for example, depends on exposure to many varied cases over a lengthy period of time.

- One crucial assumption is that doctors using the Model will subscribe fully to a patient-centred approach. **The holding thread running through our notion of expertise growth is cognitive and affective engagement with the lifeworld of the patient.** By implication it is therefore assumed, to emphasise a previous point, that a competent doctor will have the knowledge, values, attitudes and skills to gain entry to the patient's lifeworld for diagnostic, management and, where appropriate, therapeutic purposes, as listed in 'Learning outcomes for patient centred care', in the RCGP Curriculum Statement for General Practice.[21]

- Expertise growth assumes and equates to a learning process. Two learning concepts underpin consideration of a progression from competent to expert:

(i) Development of 'tacit' behaviour

Educationalists use the term 'tacit' as a means to identify when a new behaviour has been learned and practised to the point where it can be performed without conscious thinking. For example, introducing yourself to the patient, a skill introduced to first-year medical students, does not require prior thinking when a new patient enters the room. After completing 500 supervised endoscopies the physician does not normally have to think about instrument insertion. Thus, over time, various successful consulting behaviours become second nature; absorbed into a consulting skill repertoire and performed tacitly.

Expertise – expert opinion or knowledge, know-how, skill or knowledge, expertness in something (*New Shorter Oxford English Dictionary*). The 'something' in this case is family doctor consulting. Throughout *Advanced Consulting*, thinking about expertise or skill development is underpinned by the following ideas:

- ❏ expert consulting can be equated with the highest practitioner levels in other 'crafts', such as music, art, literature or theatre, in which the expertise is so well ingrained that the focus can be approached as new

- ❏ those who aspire to higher skill levels must incorporate new ideas and experiential lessons into practice repeatedly to a point when they can be performed tacitly, i.e. as a skill that occurs unconsciously, unless faced by new or problematic situations, when thinking then reverts to 'conscious'

- ❏ expertise is dependent upon the quality of experience and the quality of reflection on that experience – experience alone will not necessarily lead to growth of skill. The quality of experience may be enhanced or retarded by the organisational culture of daily practice

- ❏ practitioner performance can be tracked using the language *competent – proficient – expert* pioneered by the Dreyfus Brothers upon which the Consultation Expertise Model has been superimposed.[22]

(ii) Development of Metacognition

Closely associated with tacit behaviour is the progression from *knows* to *doing things well*, as illustrated in the adapted Miller Triangle below. Experienced professionals 'know' what to do and 'do it' automatically.[23] Indeed, it is this absence of observable, working-out behaviour that confuses professional newcomers. Experts make the task look easy and therefore difficult to copy. It is therefore necessary to add a further learning stage: the facility to reflect upon and know *what* you are doing – to be able to stand outside yourself and know, for instance, that you are *consciously* using silence to elicit what a patient really wants to say. To educators this is the process of *metacognition*.[24]

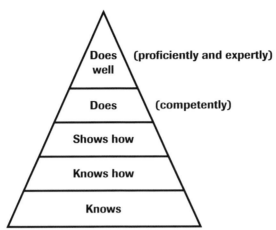

Figure 1.04 Adapted Miller Triangle

- Although the Model presents a picture of expert consulting attributes and some suggestions to assist the development of expertise, it should not be assumed to be a toolkit. It is our assumption that growth will be context-specific to particular environments and conditions and driven by individual insight and motivation – personal habits of reflection. We see our task to identify signposts across this territory, leaving the route taken through the territory to individual choice and happenstance.
- Don't for a minute think that experts consult at high levels of expertise all the time. This Model is presented by practising doctors, people whose concentration possibly does vary throughout a packed surgery, who are prone to the Friday afternoon syndrome, who do get calls to say the dog has gone through the hedge, who can be influenced by transference and counter transference; the list is endless. Performance is influenced by fallible human activity.
- We assume those reading this book will appreciate the contents to be an expression of family doctor practice situated in a particular cultural environment – expertise will always be contingent on context. That said, we believe there to be sufficient overlap of content for it to be relevant in other family doctor health worlds, perhaps with minor interpretation, as under:

An English patient went to a family doctor in Toulouse to ask for advice about a kidney infection. The doctor suggested homeopathic treatment, which is not uncommon in France. The patient agreed, having had homeopathic treatment in the UK. Based on this experience, she asked the French doctor whether she should stop drinking coffee or alcohol. The doctor, looking alarmed, replied, 'I'm sorry Madame, I seem to have given you the wrong impression, you are ill but you are not dying.'

ISSUES ARISING

The Model is *not* a summative assessment tool

When watching a consultation tape or sitting in the surgery observing and subsequently translating what's seen into a fingerprint, it is natural to think of making an assessment. Indeed, in terms of what's going on in the head, it is an assessment. We tend to get round the problem by talking about marking but that doesn't entirely avoid the problem – marking for what? Frankly, we know any model can be misused, but it is our firm belief that it would be wrong and counterproductive to use this Model for anything other than professional improvement (it must not be used punitively). **The Model has not been validated for summative assessment. It has only been validated for formative personal use.** As we intended, no two people will mark it and produce exactly the same result. If fingerprinting is followed according to the rubric, the result will be sufficiently accurate for constructive discussion. Differences in perception can be anticipated and will be the basis for dialogue.

The Model *is* complex

While some discrete aspects of the consultation may be perceived to be 'simple' or 'complicated' in that changes or replacements may improve practice, exploring the nature of consultation as a whole, as teachers are obliged to do, becomes inescapably complex. Foremost amongst the reasons for this is the fact that many family medicine encounters require unique judgements in order to deal with the uncertainty and unpredictability present in both the medicine and the characteristics of the patient. The Model is an attempt to unpack the features at work in this complex activity.

This raises two issues: one is the problem of sharing complex matters accessibly, the other of unpicking the substance of complex practice itself. Both issues surface implicitly and explicitly in what follows.

The Model *is* complicated

Some colleagues have commented that the Model presented diagrammatically looks complicated. It is. Consulting is a complex business, as we discuss on p. 131. Yet expert consulters can make the process look easy in a way that a learner may find difficult to understand. The Model captures four components of consulting expertise. These are explained in the next chapter. Each component requires sufficient detail in the description to be meaningful to a learner. Presenting these details diagrammatically is complicated but necessary so that a record of the evidence – the fingerprint – can be constructed.

The Model does not capture patient feedback

In family practice in the UK patient feedback is gathered routinely.[25]

More detailed validated questionnaires are available for learners at different levels of experience.[26,27] The relationship between consulting expertise and patient satisfaction remains to be explored however, within the Model expertise in negotiating management and achieving concordance would imply that patient satisfaction has been explicitly addressed during the consultation.

This is *not* a definitive model of expert consulting

The Model inevitably does not cover every single facet of expert consulting behaviour; for example, the Model includes no means of telling when a doctor chooses deliberately *not* to engage with an issue or problem presented in a consultation. A decision about whether to engage fully, partially or not at all permeates all consultations. Engagement raises a whole new range of fascinating questions for others to answer.

Suffice to say, components of the Model have been identified by reflecting on the group's experience in practice. As such it represents what some practitioners think happens. It can't be proved in any way other than through the approval of colleagues – others with more resource potential might be able to prove it. **It is therefore desirable that the notion of expertise in family medicine is explored further.**

References

1. Neighbour R. *The Inner Apprentice*. Dordrecht: Kluwer Academic Publishers; 1992. p. 43.
2. Sennett R. *The Craftsman*. London: Allen Lane-Penguin Books; 2008. p. 10.
3. Allen J, Rashid A. What determines competence within a general practice consultation? Assessment of consultation skills using simulated surgeries. *Br J Gen Prac*. 1998; **48**: 1259–62.
4. Pendleton D, Schofield T, Tate P, *et al*. *The New Consultation: developing doctor-patient communication*. Oxford: Oxford University Press; 2003. p. 70.
5. Tate P. *The Doctor's Communication Handbook*. 4th ed. Oxford: Radcliffe Medical Press; 2003.
6. Fraser RC. *The Leicester Assessment Package*. 2nd ed. Macclesfield: Glaxo Medical Fellowship; 1994.
7. Thew R, Worrall P. The selection and training of patient-simulators for the assessment of consultation performance in simulated surgeries. *Educ Gen Pract*. 1998; **9**(2): 211–16.

8. Norfolk T. *Developing the Personal Competencies of GP Registrars: new training modules – full report.* London: City University; 2004.
9. Norfolk T, Birdi K, Walsh D. The role of empathy in establishing rapport in the consultation: a new model. *Med Educ.* 2007; **41**: 690–7.
10. Atweh B, Kemmis S, Weeks P. *Action Research in Practice.* London: Routledge; 1998.
11. Carr W, Kemmis S. *Becoming Critical: education, knowledge and action research.* London: Falmer Press; 1986. p. 162.
12. Slobada J. Acquiring skill. In Gellatly A, editor. *The Skilful Mind: an introduction to cognitive psychology.* Milton Keynes: Open University Press; 1986. p. 33.
13. Pendleton, op cit.
14. Neighbour R. *The Inner Consultation: how to develop an effective and intuitive consulting style.* Newbury; Petroc Press; 1996.
15. Silverman J, Kurtz S, Draper J. *Skills for Communicating with Patients.* Oxford: Radcliffe Medical Press; 1998.
16. Helman C. *Culture, Health and Illness.* 4th ed. London: Hodder Arnold; 2001.
17. McWhinney I. *Textbook of Family Medicine.* Oxford: Oxford University Press; 1997.
18. Stewart M, Brown JB, Weston WW, *et al. Patient-Centred Medicine: transforming the clinical method.* Oxford: Radcliffe Medical Press; 2003.
19. Elwyn G. *Shared Decision Making: patient involvement in clinical practice.* Nijmegan: WOK; 2001.
20. Benner P. *From Novice to Expert.* NJ: Prentice Hall; 1984. p. 9.
21. RCGP. *RCGP Curriculum for General Practice: the learning and teaching guide.* London: RCGP; 2006.
22. Dreyfus H, Dreyfus S. *Mind over Machine: the power of human intuition and expertise in the era of the computer.* New York: Free Press; 1986.
23. Miller G. The Assessment of clinical skills/competence/performance. *Acad Med.* 1990; **65**: 563–7.
24. Eraut M. *Developing Professional Knowledge and Competence.* London: Falmer Press; 1994.
25. General Practice Assessment Questionnaire. Available at: www.gpaq.info/ (accessed 28 October 2008).
26. Royal College of General Practitioners. Curriculum and Assessment Site. Available at: www.rcgp-curriculum.org.uk/nmrgcp/wpba/psq.aspx (accessed 28 October 2008).
27. Evans RG, Edwards A, Evans S, *et al.* Assessing the practising physician using patient surveys: a systematic review of instruments and feedback methods. *Fam. Pract.* 2007; **24**(2): 117–27.

2 THE CONSULTATION EXPERTISE MODEL

The four components of the Consultation Expertise Model

The four components in depth
1.   Consulting skills
2.   Domains
     — The domain focus
     — An extended understanding of the domain – 'What is known'
     — A case history with a domain dominance – 'In my experience'
3.   Performance levels
4.   Indicative statements
     — The nature and purpose of indicative statements
     — A case example to illustrate use of indicative statements for marking
     — The eight domains with indicative statements and marking key
Advanced consulting – in summary

THE FOUR COMPONENTS OF THE MODEL

1. Consulting skills

Consulting skills lie at the heart of the Model. Consulting skills (as we understand them) are divided into three main areas:
1.   medical knowledge and skill
2.   clinical problem framing and solving skills
3.   interpersonal skills.

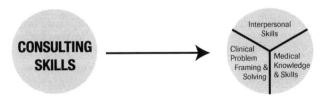

Figure 2.01 Consulting skills core

2. Domains of expertise

Expertise is described in relation to eight domains. This particular set of domains, derived from practitioner experience, has been found sufficient to reflect the range of family medical consulting practice. The eight domains are:

1. Communication
2. Recognising Patterns
3. Medical Competence
4. Respecting Patients
5. Dealing with Uncertainty
6. Use of Resources
7. Focus
8. Synthesising Skills

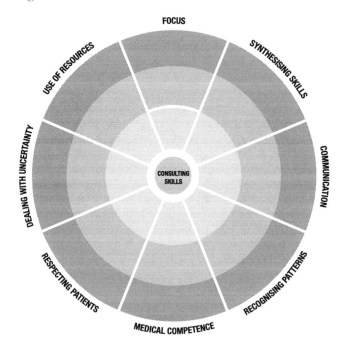

Figure 2.02 Circle with eight domains

3. Performance levels

Performance in each of the domains is represented at three levels: competent, proficient and expert.

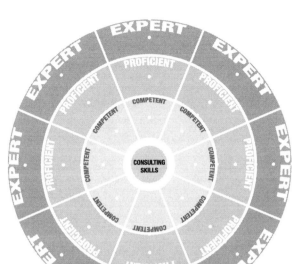

Figure 2.03 Circle with three performance levels

4. Indicative statements

Within each domain there are indicative statements for each of the three performance levels: competent, proficient and expert. Indicative statements are descriptors of observable behaviour. They provide the doctor with the means to associate actions they have witnessed with levels of performance, thus enabling them to provide evidence for a judgement on their own or a colleague's stage of consulting.

We will now consider the meaning invested in each of these four components and their implications for practice.

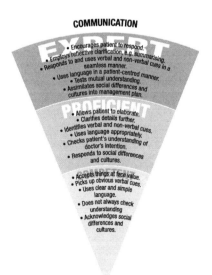

Figure 2.04 Indicative statements for Communication domain

WHAT WE MEAN BY – CONSULTING SKILLS

The notion of consulting skills at the centre of the Model is predicated first on the individuality and professional training of each family practitioner; second on expertise development in three core skill fields; and third on the belief that performance can change holistically over time to deliver higher-level outcomes in practice.

Though consulting skills may not develop systematically, they can and will change and become more effective over time for most family doctors. The Consultation Expertise Model is presented on the understanding that, although consultation skills are not evaluated directly in the Model, they provide the means by which domain performance and expertise can be tracked. A clarifying question may, for example, reinforce rapport at the same time as negotiating uncertainty. Interpersonal skill observations may well be disclosed explicitly in the post-consultation analysis and will inevitably figure in feedback discussions. Consulting skills should be considered to underpin and be integrated into the behaviours identified in the Model.

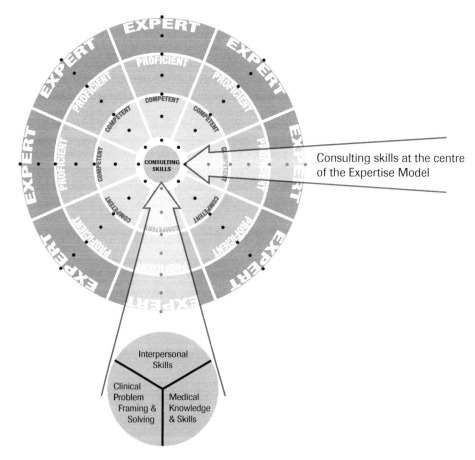

Figure 2.05 Consulting skills – essential skills at the core of the Model

'The essential unit of medical practice is the occasion when, in the intimacy of the consulting room, or the sick room, a person who is ill or believes himself to be ill, seeks the advice of a doctor whom he trusts. This is a consultation and all else in medicine derives from it.'[1]

> Consulting skills are understood uniquely by each family doctor.

It is necessary to ask why there is a need to explain what is meant by the term 'consulting skills'. Surely for practising doctors it goes without saying; everyone has their own unique understanding of what consulting skills are.

However, it's not sufficient (nor particularly helpful) to leave this implicit understanding and move on, as we need to explain how consulting skills function in the context of the Model and furthermore, how they can be expressed at an expert level.

> Consulting skills operate uniquely and differently at expert level.

There are three key components to consulting skills:
1. medical knowledge and skill
2. clinical problem framing and solving skills
3. interpersonal skills.

Each can be looked at from the point of view of:
- the **language** used to explore the nature of high-level consulting skill
- pointers as to how **doctors may learn** to develop expertise in order to achieve high levels of skill
- illustrations of the **professional application** of these skills through real-life case examples.

> As consulting experience grows, the core skills repertoire becomes more crafted.

The view taken here is that consulting skill in family medicine is based on an amalgam of these three specialised skilled fields interacting with one another. Though separated here, it is the interplay of these skills that gives rise to that all-important quality, patient trust. However, this breaks no new ground; it merely extracts core elements from clinical method and internationally available models of good practice that are compatible with *The European Definition of General Practice/ Family Medicine*[2] and, more recently, the Royal College of General Practice (RCGP) Curriculum Statement.[3]

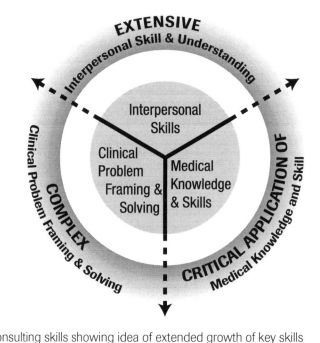

Figure 2.06 Consulting skills showing idea of extended growth of key skills

Medical knowledge and skill

'The relationship between the body of scientific knowledge and the skilled practice of a general practitioner in their surgery is extremely complex.'[4]

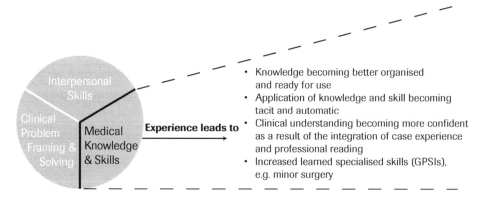

Figure 2.07 Critical application of medical knowledge and skills – features of skill development

Learning to develop expertise in medical knowledge and skill

The four aspects of medical knowledge and skill in Figure 2.07, chosen to illustrate a notion of what experienced consulters do, cannot normally be achieved by new doctors because, by implication, the outcomes selected are dependent on years of experience. It is self-evident that new formally learned skills, such as minor surgery, will improve performance. There is research evidence to support the manner in which secure knowledge impacts on confidence, the way knowledge is used more effectively (and efficiently) with experience and, as a consequence, the way that responses become quicker and more automatic. This process is sometimes referred to as 'automatisation'[5] but here the more neutral word 'tacit' is preferred – Polanyi invented the term 'tacit knowledge' to describe that which we know but cannot tell.[6]

> With increased experience comes a more immediate and skilled application of medical knowledge and skill.

'Finally, the "experienced GP" has a condensed set of information about defined "problem groups". In their minds GPs combine pathophysiology, symptoms and therapy within a certain context in one global set of linked information. These are called scripts.'[7]

CASE EXAMPLE: PROFESSIONAL APPLICATION OF MEDICAL KNOWLEDGE AND SKILLS

I observed my registrar, who was early on in his family doctor placement but quite an experienced doctor, consulting with a 28-year-old woman who was about seven weeks pregnant. He'd already started the process of trying to find out what might be going on. She might be bleeding – might have problems. She had abdominal pain. He'd quite quickly come up with two or three possible diagnoses. Top of his list was a urine infection. He'd thought about bowel problems but ruled those out fairly quickly. He wondered about an ectopic pregnancy. The problem-solving issue ran through it. The urine specimen was positive.

He examined her and found that the pain was higher than you would have expected for an ectopic pregnancy. So he reduced that down his list of priorities. Then there was the question of how to approach the problem of an ectopic pregnancy with her, just in case. He told me he'd ruled it out given the history and the examination but the patient herself said she wondered whether there were any other possible causes. The question was how to frame it for her in terms of what was most likely and what conditions it was important not to miss. He said, 'We are fairly sure that it is a urine infection, for which we'll give you some treatment . . . but if it doesn't go away, or if this happens or that happens, you must come straight back – though we've ruled it out, we can never be 100% certain. It was a case of framing it for her. She made it easy for him by being bright and well read. She fed him the lines. It would have been a harder process with a less keen-to-know patient, without frightening her.

The higher skill is framing it for the patient. If you can't frame it for yourself then you can't frame it for the patient. You have to go back one and ask yourself, 'What am I thinking?' There are things you shouldn't miss. A renal stone could have been on that list from where the pain was but that got ruled out fairly quickly on testing the urine, as you would expect to get blood there. You can only frame clearly and safely if you know your medicine.

Clinical problem framing and solving

> *'Experience . . . does not refer to the mere passage of time or longevity. Rather, it is the refinement of preconceived notions and theory through encounters with many actual practical situations that add nuances or shades of differences to theory.'*[8]

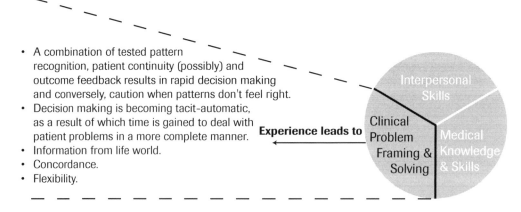

- A combination of tested pattern recognition, patient continuity (possibly) and outcome feedback results in rapid decision making and conversely, caution when patterns don't feel right.
- Decision making is becoming tacit-automatic, as a result of which time is gained to deal with patient problems in a more complete manner.
- Information from life world.
- Concordance.
- Flexibility.

Experience leads to Clinical Problem Framing & Solving

Interpersonal Skills

Medical Knowledge & Skills

Figure 2.08 Complex clinical problem framing and solving skills

Learning to develop expertise in medical problem framing and solving
The later expansion on problem framing (*see* p. 144) provides an explanation of how helpful it is to draw a distinction between initial *problem framing* and *problem solving* underpinning management decisions.

> *'. . . theories of clinical decision making by physicians. These are more strongly linked to research evidence (EBM), yet encompass both intuitive models based on memory and analytic models based on probabilities and reasoning.'*[9]

All the features illustrating how changes in problem framing and solving define higher levels of expertise in Figure 2.08 have been chosen because they each, again by implication, require significant periods of experience to achieve.

> 'Pattern recognition is associated with 10 fold greater odds of diagnostic success than using hypothetico-deductive reasoning. The aptitude to exploit this strategy occurs with expertise and its use by medical students is not advocated because of potentially dire consequences.'[10]

> With experience, problem framing and solving becomes quicker and more secure.

Completeness, a feature of the expert consultation and an outcome of a holistic approach, is only possible if full account of bio-psycho-social information is included in the problem framing. This requires engagement with the patient's agenda and lifeworld but enables greater understanding both by and with the patient. Completeness thus influences the use and effectiveness of resources (*see* Concordance, p.158). **The extent to which decisions are shared is itself a function of higher-order expertise.**

> 'Paternalism, informed choice and shared decision making are the terms now commonly used to describe the spectrum of patient involvement in decision making.'[11]

CASE EXAMPLE: PROFESSIONAL APPLICATION OF CLINICAL PROBLEM FRAMING AND SOLVING SKILLS

I saw a lady – before I go any further I think it is important to say, when you get to the cause of a problem and you are the fourth or fifth doctor in a line, it doesn't mean that you are the best doctor in the line. Often what's been done before has allowed the picture to be framed or things have progressed to such an extent that it's now clear; for instance, if you see somebody with a rash and you make the diagnosis and they have seen four other people with the rash, it can be that the rash did not show its pathognomonic features before they got to you. The patient often says 'I wish I had seen you in the first place'. Actually, I wouldn't have got it if she had.

This is a lady who came in to see me with a combination of features that could point either to the menopause or depression. But her presenting feature originally had been being tired all the time – she had seen a doctor about that and had been investigated and nothing had been found. There had been a further discussion about the menopause with another doctor and a discussion about depression with yet another doctor. When she came to see me I had the advantage of knowing that each of those had really not hit. Discussing what had happened so far and where it had got her, I had one of those flash moments when you think – 'OK I'm going to try something here'. I consciously thought how to introduce it, because it's a tricky topic. One of my medical school professors used to say that many menopausal symptoms weren't treatable with HRT because they have 'empty nest syndrome'. Take someone who has a wonderful torrid courtship, they are in love, then they get married and the marriage changes to a new level of relationship. The children come along and then, coincidently around the time of the menopause, the children leave home or don't need the parents any longer. The parents haven't reformed their relationship and it can seem (this may be stereotyping) that many women suffer from empty nest syndrome.

It was just the way this lady was talking – so rather than say to her, 'I think you have got empty nest syndrome', which may seem pejorative, I actually said, 'Well I was taught by this professor who used to say . . . and then ran through it with her. She burst into tears and said, 'You have hit the nail on the head, that's been the reason that I have been feeling like this.'

And we talked it through a bit and she went off and agreed to come and see me in a while once she'd reflected on it. She came back and said, 'My husband and I have talked and we both think that you are the first one who has listened to me.' I said, 'No, I'm not. I had the advantage of all the previous consultations and all I did was reflect back what I thought you were telling me.'

Interpersonal skills

> '. . . the importance of forming a human relationship between doctor and patient . . . is the basis of good consulting, and it requires the ability to identify imaginatively with what a patient experiences subjectively during an illness, and to recognise the validity and importance of that experience for the patient.'[12]

Learning to develop expertise in interpersonal skills

> A wider repertoire of interpersonal skill combines with increasingly perceptive patient relationships.

Skill, according to the Dreyfus brothers, is 'an integrative overarching approach to professional action.'[13]

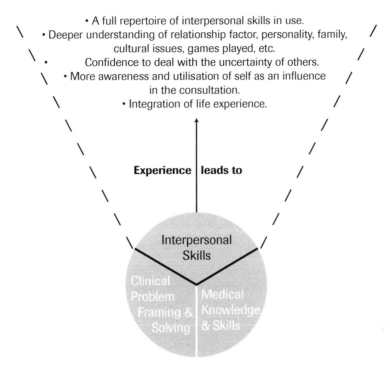

Figure 2.09 Extended interpersonal skills

> *In order to be good doctors, we need to be scientists with our minds and artists*
> *with our hearts – corrupted Chinese proverb*

In many ways this is the most engaging developmental area of the three. It is much less technical and knowledge bound and yet potentially the key to higher-level expertise. In many cases, interpersonal skill opens the door to more complete history-taking, to the melding of biomedical and biographical aspects of a case, to achieving concordance and (as those who have explored the use of paintings and literature have found) the possibility of more creative consulting. There is much to be said for considering expert consulting as an art.

> *'. . . while there is a large and profoundly important scientific element in the*
> *practice of medicine, there is also an indefinable artistry, an imaginative insight,*
> *and medicine (they will tell us) is born of a marriage between the two.'*[14]

Artists in this sense are practitioners who have mastered their trade to such an extent that they can consider different forms of application and interpretation.

The case narrative of an experienced doctor consulting with Judith Anderson – a patient simulation of an older woman trapped in an unloving marriage and burdened with unresolved medical issues – provides a good example of creative interpretation. This is explained more fully in the feedback section later (*see* p. 116). Having listened to Mrs Anderson's complicated story and current problems, the doctor afterwards discloses that he was privately likening her condition to that of a caged bird. Fanciful maybe, but the metaphor was crucial to his decision making. Could he risk what might happen if his management plan opened the door of the cage? Or, the effect of a too-abrupt change of style?

> '. . . talking does not necessarily change one's own or other people's feelings or ideas. I believe the 21st century needs a new ambition, to develop not talk but conversation, which does change people. Real conversation catches fire. It involves more than sending and receiving information.'[15]

As responses to medical problems become tacit[16] it becomes possible to pay more attention to the person of the patient, to converse in a more relaxed manner and gradually become more perceptive of the way patients behave. Whether through life experience (one recalls the young male doctor floundering over the treatment of nappy rash) or through reading, our understanding of people and ourselves (what we bring to the consultation), the chemistry of the interaction, becomes more 'knowing' over time. Just how it happens is difficult to say, but the use of interpersonal skills seems to expand both in range and quality. One can expect cues to be picked up during early training, but the more subtle clues sensed from pauses, changes in tone, half spoken disclosures or shifts in body language, what one colleague referred to as 'the music of the consultation', may not be. These require a level of attention only possible from a doctor who, with greater self-knowledge, has fine-tuned their radar.

In terms of an interpersonal skill repertoire, it is noticeable when looking at video tapes that experienced doctors use a greater number of identifiable skills, as well as adapting and extending the effectiveness of basic skills such as listening, use of silence and questioning. This must be achieved by the doctor as self-learner because, 'for behaviour to be regarded as skilled, it must have been learned'.[17] We also know these advanced behaviours are not likely to be the result of formal learning: post certification there is no standard programme for the development of interpersonal skills.

CASE EXAMPLE: PROFESSIONAL APPLICATION OF INTERPERSONAL SKILLS

She is a patient with recurrent depression. Her last episode was over a year ago. This current episode is triggered by increasing work stress. She knows the signs and symptoms, so she came knowing what the problem was. She responded previously to a combination of counselling and medication. The consultation allowed us to talk a little bit more deeply about what was going on at work because that seemed to be the key stressor. Although she had dealt with some of the issues about 18 months earlier, things were escalating for her, and based on the fact that we have known each other for a number of years, and based on the fact that previously we had had a reasonably successful result, she seemed prepared to talk in greater depth about what was going on at work. She was feeling let down by her colleagues, colleagues she'd had working relationships with for about 20 years. There was a sense of being bullied by other members of the team. That seemed to have become worse in the last 12 months. I got a sense she was baring her soul a little bit more – her mental state allowed her to be a bit more open this time round.

It was partly trust and not having to go over the superficial details. I knew that she had a supportive family – but interestingly they work within psychiatric circles. She doesn't want to feel cornered by the family so I'm more of an independent referee – listening and encouraging her to delve a little bit deeper – almost challenging her to think of the trigger factors, particularly at work – giving her permission to get upset within the consultation, which she did.

I am conscious of sitting back in my chair, and in my work I get through a lot of tissues. I turn away from the computer and the desk and overstate my 'I have time' demeanour. Then I ask more probing, hopefully self-revealing, future-looking questions. As a result she has very much taken charge of the work situation. She has addressed it with her line managers and she is having a temporary secondment to another department. From her perspective it's not a running-away move – in her department she had felt that she had been getting the blame for everything.

Other influences on the consultation

> 'Diversity is the key to understanding complex systems. It can be seen in the many agents or influences that may affect a consultation. Some agents are physically present including the doctor, patient, and others, such as a nurse or relative . . . [it's] suggested the manager, lawyer, statistician, journalist, and computer have agency within a consultation. Their agency is through those individuals physically present.'[18]

There are of course many other influences on the consultation, some local, some national. These are real influences affecting what happens between patient and doctor, imperatives that come from practice policies, funding agencies, media scares and so on. Indeed, amongst these external pressures, the computer has almost become a third person in the room; an intruder that demands to be managed with additional skills.

However important such factors may be from time to time, we consider the three areas of professional skill above to operate on a higher plane of importance than other influences.

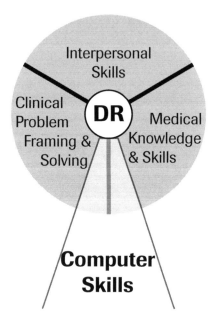

Figure 2.10 The computer – symbol of the external world

The doctor in the consultation

But let's stop for a moment. If we are to unpack our understanding of what we mean by consulting skills from scratch, aren't we missing something vital – the person of the doctor, the 'I' in the consultation – the 'professional self'?[19] After all, consulting is so unique, so dependent upon the personality, the professional values and increasingly the will to learn of each consultant that surely the doctor should be at the very centre of the consulting skills circle.

While we can explore the development potential of the three consulting skills mentioned above (medical knowledge and skill, clinical problem framing and solving skills and interpersonal skills), the development dynamic resides with the unique 'I' or 'me' in the consultation. It is not intended here to explore important doctor variables such as motivation, self-awareness or professional principles and values. Nevertheless, it would be a curiously abstract model that airbrushes out one of the main players while placing such emphasis on interactive behaviours; particularly so in a profession that is totally reliant on the skill and integrity of the individual.

> More than capability and personality is invested in the person of the doctor.

In the context of the Model it needs to be appreciated that the way family doctors consult reflects the various approaches, aspirations and templates that come under the general heading of consultation models in whatever manner each doctor has responded to them. This is of crucial importance because the Consultation Expertise Model needs to be seen as a way of looking at existing family practice, not as some new bright idea. So the person of the doctor at the core of our consultation thinking embodies not only the professional persona of the doctor, but also an awareness of what constitutes good family practice. This is a necessary presumption for doctors considered to be competent in this Model.

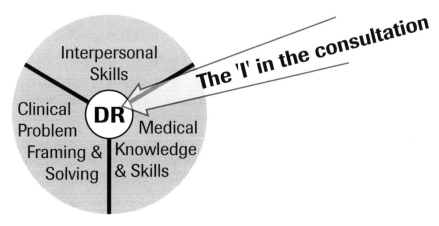

Figure 2.11 The most important consulting skills variable

The diagrams above (Figures 2.06–2.11) still only represent a one-dimensional starting point. A diagrammatic sense of movement is required to accompany the progression represented in the Model by the three performance levels. This is because the Consultation Expertise Model is predicated on the growth of consulting skills in parallel with and in support of the growth of clinical expertise. Indeed, consulting skills are seen as the means by which expert clinical behaviours are acted out.

As skills develop and change over time, it is important to have some idea of how the three skills change in their linked development with the growth of clinical expertise. In practice we see these core consulting skills becoming more integrated and sophisticated. As performance becomes more integrated, core skills become difficult to detect. Learning theorists who focus on professional skill development, such as Michael Eraut,[20] state that intended behaviour change becomes second nature with repetition, i.e. becomes tacit and therefore happens without conscious reasoning. It also happens sequentially as extended skills, i.e. deeper levels of the existing skills, are absorbed into the professional repertoire. So it becomes necessary to consider consulting skills *dynamically* in order to emphasise the crucial role

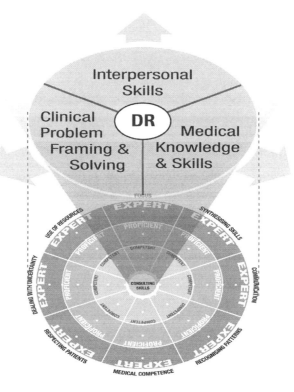

Figure 2.12 Consulting skills developing in parallel with clinical performance

that increasingly sophisticated consulting skills play in developing clinical expertise.

> Expertise in the three consultation skill components develops in parallel with clinical expertise and becomes the means whereby expert consulting is expressed.

CASE EXAMPLE

A chap came in a couple of weeks back. He'd been in a day or two before with a non-specific illness. The moment he walked through the door I knew he'd got a rash called erythema multiforme, a classical pattern – there was nothing else it could be [medical knowledge]. And therefore it meant going back into the depths of my memory – which things cause erythema multiforme? – how do I act on those? – what do I say to him? – what do I investigate? – what treatments do I give? [knowledge gaps]. The consultation was based around pattern recognition. Then I had to apply the knowledge [problem framing]. The skill is in talking through with him the possible causes and explaining, 'When I said to you erythema multiforma, your eyes went up – it sounds like a bad condition – but it just means a multi-shaped red rash.'

The knowledge was – that's what he has got – but what does that mean for him? How am I going to manage him [interpersonal skill] – the skill was in verbalising all that towards an agreed understanding.

DOMAINS OF EXPERTISE
Communication

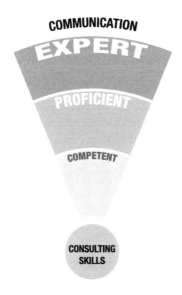

Figure 2.13 Communication – domain segment

Communication is dependent upon the use of wide and extended interpersonal skills and skilled behaviours. The intuitive, focused doctor will be able to listen more intently, while alert to cues and clues. With his/her attention freed and with his/her ability to notice and recognise patterns, the expert doctor is better equipped to read subtext, sense verbal and non-verbal cues and interpret transactions.

Meanwhile, assessment of the *doctor's own feelings* can be used as a diagnostic tool. This ability also enables him/her to modify his own responses. Using language and behaviour tailored to his/her patient's cultural, social, emotional and intellectual status, s/he can reinforce his/her verbal response with non-verbal signals, creating atmosphere and mood appropriate to his/her patient's presentation. S/he is likely to generate more interactive dialogue, testing mutual understanding and stimulating response from his patient, creating a deeper level of negotiation leading to greater concordance.

COMMUNICATION – WHAT IS KNOWN

- There is no shortage of published instruction, guidance and exhortation as to what *ought* to take place during the doctor–patient interaction. But for family doctors in full-time practice, finding out how best to communicate with patients occurs as a consequence of actually seeing patients.
- The communication ability to elicit, respond, explain, inform, negotiate and conclude is achieved through the interplay of questioning, listening, empathising, use of silence, recognising verbal and non-verbal cues and clues and the use of suitable language and demeanour – the interpersonal skills.
- Pattern recognition extends beyond the clinical to embrace recognition of patient characteristics and psycho-social factors.
- A significant percentage of emotion is conveyed non-verbally.

A young woman attended the Out of Hours Co-op on Saturday afternoon with a history of headache, stiff neck and photophobia but looked quite well. I wondered why she had come, thinking she was probably concerned about meningitis with those symptoms. I was surprised when she said she'd come because her boyfriend thought she might be pregnant. If I'd not asked for her ideas, concerns etc., I'd never have thought of that diagnosis for those symptoms and she would have left unhappy.

- The experienced doctor uses a range of 'extended' interpersonal skills, just as master craftsmen pick up brushes, tools or an instrument to create something new. An example of an 'extended' interpersonal skill might be as simple, or as profound, as a quietly suggested, 'there's more to it isn't there?'
- Communication at higher levels is driven by personal values and professional beliefs such as those invested in patient-centred consulting and shared decision making.

  'The desire reflects motivation; the ability reflects skills.'[21]

  'The bridge between teller and listener of a (patient) story turns out not only to carry traffic in both directions, but to carry multiple levels of traffic as well.'[22]

- Communication is what happens on *the bridge* at different levels.

AT A SIMULATED PATIENT WORKSHOP WITH FAMILY DOCTORS IN TRAINING – A PATIENT'S STORY

(Doctors have outline notes indicating that the patient's only daughter, whose husband happens to be a teetotaller, has been in touch with the surgery on several occasions expressing concern that her mother has been drinking a bottle of sherry a day. Offers to babysit have become an issue because of worries about the children's safety.)

I simulate a 58-year-old widow (who looks older). My husband died 10 years ago, leaving me well-off. Three years ago I was admitted to hospital with gallstones and told I have pancreatitis and must stop drinking alcohol. I am not sure what pancreatitis is but I am sure that a little drink won't do me any harm. I come to the doctors with bad stomach ache which I've had on and off for some time.

Doctors soon establish that the stomach ache is linked to the pancreatitis, though I never admit to having more than a sociable drink with my friends. During group discussion, I often hear about the likely 'bad news' factor. Invariably, every effort is made to make me admit how much I drink. On occasions the daughter's telephone calls are mentioned. This makes me angry as I am ashamed of my drinking. Once and only once, a doctor who'd been watching various attempts to make me confess came and sat by me. Very quietly he looked at me and said, 'Life has not been easy for you has it – you've been having a rough time.' And it all came out. I burst into tears and told him all about it, even where I hide the empty bottles. He didn't have to ask any questions.

- Empathy used skilfully can be very powerful.

  'The really important selling point is simple: effective communication is essential to the practice of high-quality medicine.'[23]

  'When anyone speaks to me, I listen more to the tonal modulation in his voice than to what he is actually saying. From this I know at once what he is like, what he feels, whether he is lying, whether he is agitated or whether he is merely making conventional conversation. I can even feel, or rather hear, any hidden sorrow. Life is sound, the tonal modulations of human speech. Every living creation is filled with the deepest truth. That you see has been one of the main needs of my life.'[24]

COMMUNICATION – IN MY EXPERIENCE

NECK PAIN

A consultant physician I know of the old school told me of a woman patient with neck pain who he'd been seeing every six months for many years. Every time she came he tried something else and what's more, she was seeing her family doctor in the meantime. After a few years, as she was leaving the consulting room he had a flash of inspiration and shouted after her 'Who is the pain in your neck'? She replied 'My husband'. Very soon her neck pain resolved.

THE NOTHING-SAID CONSULTATION

I was told by a family doctor, who was about to retire, of a consultation where he had not spoken during the entire consultation. I remember him telling me this as a family doctor trainee and me being rather horrified. He hadn't used any of the skills that we were being taught. He hadn't explored her ideas, concerns and expectations etc. A while ago I found myself in a similar situation. A patient who was well known to me came in and told me what she had come about and proceeded to analyse and discuss this with herself. With appropriate nods and noises of encouragement from me she reached the end of the consultation, thanked me for my help and got up and left before I had a chance to say anything.

The family doctor who I thought was appalling when he told me this story is now my patient, so I took much pleasure in telling him.

Recognising Patterns

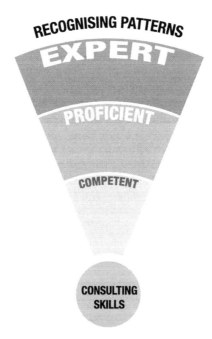

Figure 2.14 Recognising Patterns – domain segment

The skill domain most directly relating to the theory of expertise is that of pattern recognition, which is fundamental to the development of intuitive judgement. The patterns that experienced doctors recognise include cues and clues in verbal and non-verbal communication; neuro-linguistic behaviour patterns; emotional, cultural, social and transactional patterns; and clusters of physical signs and syndromes of symptoms and their severity.

It is possible, with reasonable certainty, to discriminate when a consulter has identified a diagnostic, emotional or behaviour pattern. This can be inferred from the route taken in the ensuing consultation and might be verified from the subsequent doctor's or patient's narrative. Of course, some doctors probably recognise patterns, cues and clues subliminally, and so might not be sufficiently aware of their own observations to describe them in a case narrative, but so long as they have enough confidence in their intuition to test out these clues, then proficient or expert behaviour might be inferred.

RECOGNISING PATTERNS – WHAT IS KNOWN

- Pattern recognition often appears both easy and fast in expert consulters – this is because reasoning has become fluent and *intuitive*.
- Previous encounters and interactions with the patient or scenario will shape practitioners' reasoning.

I watched a GPR recording of a perfectly competent clinical exchange with a 16-year-old and his mother. He had a sore throat and earache and a possible allergy. The registrar agreed with the patient's theory that he may well be allergic to horses, which is why his eyes were swollen and he had a blotchy rash round his face when he rubbed his eyes – having stroked a horse. He also had a past history of bad earaches and he had a bit of a red eardrum. So medically very competent – covered all the bases – the big question I had at the end of that consultation was, 'Why had that patient come?' With an allergy that was recognised and an earache for which this 16-year-old had been regularly treated, one wonders why they came today – what was the patient's agenda? Maybe there were two agendas! Here was an illustration of an incomplete pattern.

- Conclusions are reached by *clinical intuition* and analytical reasoning which is largely based on *probability and factual data*. At times these may conflict, requiring further exploration of the level of *congruency* of what you are seeing and hearing with what you are feeling.

A man in his late sixties came to evening surgery. I know him well, though he presents infrequently, usually with minor problems. His opening words were, 'I want something for my tummy.' I went into the history and it became clear he was describing a pain which came on with exercise, not related to eating and relieved by rest. On examination I found him to be hypertensive and also to have a heart murmur. An ECG showed that he had ischemic heart disease. He was referred and found to have aortic stenosis. He had heart valve surgery and was treated for his hypertension. This all stemmed from recognising that his pain was not due to a GI problem but of ischemic heart disease in nature.

I was pleased I recognised the pattern of the pain he was describing and avoided jumping to the patient's interpretation of his pain.

● As there is potential for reasoning to be coloured by previous experience with a similar situation or experience, a practitioner needs to be wary that they may become overly committed to a particular hypothesis, e.g. power of labelling or assumptions.

I had a case recently where I missed a diagnosis of a pituitary tumour in a young Iraqi man who was a failed asylum seeker. He had been presenting with recurrent headaches and feeling generally unwell. Because of his complicated personal and social circumstances, I had concluded that his symptoms were due to stress and I had been treating him accordingly until his condition acutely worsened and necessitated hospital admission.

On reflection I realised how intuition-driven my actions had been. I have dealt with many failed asylum seekers before who often present with stress and anxiety-related headaches. My diagnosis in this case was largely based on assumptions derived from previous pattern recognition. Subsequently my pattern recognition has needed to change to accommodate further 'patterns' for patients presenting with headaches. The process of pattern recognition is always dynamic and is constantly evolving.

> 'It is likely that experienced practitioners use a hypothetico-deductive strategy only with difficult cases. Diagnostic accuracy does not depend as much on strategy but more on mastery of content. Whether a diagnostic problem is deemed difficult or not is resultant on the practitioner's experience and knowledge.'[25]

> 'To be a successful decision maker, we have to edit. The answer is that our unconscious engages in "thin slicing", which is a critical component of rapid cognition. "Thin slicing" refers to the ability of our unconscious to find patterns in situations and behaviour based on very narrow slices of experience. Our internal computer effortlessly and instantly finds a pattern in chaos. If we could not thin-slice and make sense of complicated situations in a flash, driving, for example, would be chaotic!'[26]

● Pattern recognition extends beyond the clinical to embrace recognition of patient characteristics and psycho-social factors.
● Pattern recognition is idiosyncratic.

> '. . . because of different experiences, different physicians may develop different scripts [patterns] for the same disease. In other words, the scripts are

highly idiosyncratic and bear only superficial relationship to the descriptions of 'prototypical' cases as they appear in clinical textbooks.'[27]

- Pattern recognition is inextricably linked to quality of experience.

RECOGNISING PATTERNS – IN MY EXPERIENCE

Our appointment system changed and I found myself dealing with acute cases, a lot of patients with flu. After a few days it struck me that I was able to identify symptoms before they were mentioned. The patient only needed to give me one or two key features and it was enough for me to recognise the particular strain of the virus going round. This particular flu seemed to start with vomiting. Many got a pounding headache and chest pains they described as 'wanting to hold their chest as if their chest was exploding'. This was the kind of language they actually used. I found myself able to identify more or less what they had with a degree of accuracy. This allowed me to limit my history-taking and spend longer on management and other things because I was fairly confident I was making the right diagnosis, as I had become aware of an emerging pattern.

Medical Competence

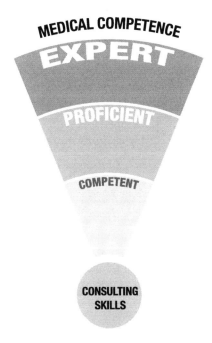

Figure 2.15 Medical Competence – domain segment

However empathic and receptive a doctor may be, s/he is not effective unless applying sound, evidence-based, scientific medicine. But expertise involves more than simply having enough medical knowledge to practise safely. Even the most expert consulter has gaps in his/her knowledge or is unsure of the quality of that knowledge or the judgements made. The skill involves knowing how to apply this knowledge, having the ability to assess the quality of personal knowledge and judgement, identifying possible weaknesses and creating strategies for addressing them. Involving the patient in this process permits them both to share the reasoning towards diagnosis or management plans and negotiate or challenge the quality of judgements made.

MEDICAL COMPETENCE – WHAT IS KNOWN

- Medical Competence requires understanding and application of evidence-based medicine (EBM) with regard to patients' values and beliefs.

  'EBM is not "cookbook" medicine. Because it requires a bottom-up approach that integrates the best of external evidence with individual clinical expertise and patients' choice, it cannot result in slavish, cookbook approaches to individual patient care. External clinical evidence can inform, but never replace, individual clinical expertise, and it is this expertise that decides whether the external evidence applies to the individual patient at all and, if so, how it should be integrated into a clinical decision. Similarly, any external guideline must be integrated with individual clinical expertise in deciding whether and how it matches the patient's clinical state, predicament and preferences, and thus whether it should be applied. Clinicians who fear top-down cookbooks will find the advocates of EBM joining them at the barricades.'[28]

- The application of clinical knowledge and skill, modified in response to patient circumstances, may lie within the domain of Synthesising Skills.

  'Doctors conduct an inner consultation with biomedical evidence before deciding how to apply it.'[29]

- The ability to apply medical understanding (doctor agenda) to the patient's agenda requires a step beyond the confines of a purely biomedical agenda, i.e. 'going there' (*see* p. 156).[30]
- There is an implication that Medical Competence requires working with the truth. Inevitably, this introduces the possibility of confrontation or ethical dilemmas.

The following story indicates this aspect of consulting:

'The patient had a long-standing and refractory clinical depression and had tried most of the available antidepressants without effect until she was enrolled in a drug trial. The new treatment gave her dramatic and sustained improvement, much to the relief of her clinical caregivers. However, she had, in fact, been on the placebo arm of the trial. As ethicist, I was asked what her treating clinicians should tell her.'[31]

- The required medical skills are set out in *Good Medical Practice*, GMC, paragraphs 2–14, November 2006.[32]
- Medical Competence requires professional confidence and self-awareness gained through experience. So a new entrant might be clinically highly competent but not be medically competent in the sense we use it here.
- Medical Competence as applied in the Consultation Expertise Model goes beyond being medically up to date; it is about how medical 'know-how' is applied.

MEDICAL COMPETENCE – IN MY EXPERIENCE

A 43-year-old woman attended surgery four days after a bout of sickness and diarrhoea. She was seen by a partner, fully examined and told she had a post-viral illness. She re-attended three days later with symptoms of dysuria and on examination she was tender super-pubically and in a renal angle.

However, an MSU showed no evidence of infection. She didn't respond to antibiotics and came back three days later looking and feeling worse. She felt extremely tired and had quite marked pelvic pain. When I did a vaginal examination she had an extremely tender uterus. However, this did not seem to be a standard cervical excitation linked to pelvic inflammatory disease – I had never seen anything like this before. She was apyrexial but tachycardic. She was fairly acutely unwell but I didn't feel she warranted an immediate referral to hospital. She herself was unwilling to go into hospital. Nevertheless, I wondered if this was something obscure like a pyometria or endometritis and discussed it with the duty gynaecology doctor. We agreed that she didn't warrant urgent admission at 4.30pm that afternoon. However I safety-netted and said if she became more unwell she could go into the gynae ward overnight. An ultrasound scan was organised for her the next morning.

I told her very carefully what to do during the night if she became unwell. She and her husband were happy with the safety netting and were very clear about the steps to take. She told me she was very grateful to be able to stay at home in her own bed.

Comment – The doctor in this case framed a management plan rather than a diagnosis and avoided using resources without benefit to the patient.

Respecting Patients

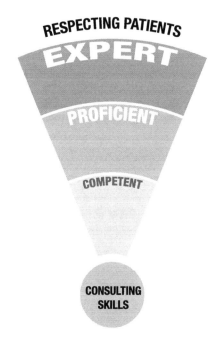

Figure 2.16 Respecting Patients – domain segment

Increased communication skills give the expert doctor a greater understanding of how patients' problems affect their lives. They enhance the ability to see and feel patients' perspectives, particularly from their cultural, social and intellectual position. Improved expressive communication skills allow the doctor to adapt his/her way of working so as to be understandable and acceptable to patients whatever their standpoint.

There is another element to respecting patients, however, that does not flow naturally from experience and developing expertise. In order to use these skills to full effect, an ethical dimension is added; it is the willingness to value patients for who they are in their own terms.

With these skills the doctor and patient can relate more equally and the doctor can work with the individuality of patients, their aspirations, constraints, beliefs and past experience. The problem can then be dealt with in the context of the patient's whole life, encompassing both inner and external environments.

RESPECTING PATIENTS – WHAT IS KNOWN

- Outcomes can be influenced when the *lifeworld* is included in the consultation.

'When doctor and patient engaged with the lifeworld, more of the agenda was voiced (Mutual Lifeworld) and patients were recognized as unique human beings (psychological plus physical problems). Poorest outcomes occurred where patients used the voice of the lifeworld but were ignored (Lifeworld Blocked) by doctors' use of the voice of medicine (chronic physical complaints).'[33]

'The analysis supports the premise that increased use of the lifeworld makes for better outcomes and more humane treatment of patients as unique human beings.'[34]

- Working with the individuality of the patient affects outcomes.

It might be useful to think of *respecting patients* in terms of levels.

Every-person level: Attitudes to people in general, i.e. warmth, values, ethical standpoints, views on equity, customary interpersonal behaviour etc.

Professional level: Best described in Carl Rogers' phrase as giving 'unconditional positive regard'. That is, showing professional regard for patients irrespective of personal feelings.*

Eliciting level: Establishing the patient's agenda, ideas, concerns and expectations but not overtly dealing with them.

Engaging level: Discussing the patient's problem in terms of their lifeworld. Using lifeworld knowledge and emotion to formulate a management plan.

Concordant level: Explicitly negotiating an agreed management plan. This agreement might respect the patient's position to the extent of overriding the doctors declared best plan.

Therapeutic level: The doctor takes face-to-face action in assisting the patient to deal with anxiety, distress and other health inhibiting conditions by conversational means.

*'For there to be interpersonal congruence between doctor and patient, the doctor should be exactly what he or she is without façade, role or pretence.'[35]

● Doctors' use of patients' ideas in negotiated decision making can be improved.

'. . . future developments in this area (shared decision making) depend on increasing the time available within consultations, require improved ways of communicating risk to patients and an acquisition of new communication skills.'[36]

● Patient complaints are frequently located at the 'every-person level'.

'Doctors who treat patients disrespectfully or delivered information insensitively and inadequately were far more likely to end up in court.'[37]

RESPECTING PATIENTS – IN MY EXPERIENCE

I am thinking about an Asian woman who presented with schizophrenia, so for me there were two factors to engage with. The first, her schizophrenia, manifested itself peculiarly in that she was Hindu but with a Muslim woman living inside of her. Her delusion was of the woman inside her. And the second issue in regard to showing respect for her was both cultural and linguistic. I don't speak Hindi or Gujarati, whereas she speaks fragmented English and thinks she speaks better English than she does. Furthermore she insists on not using a translator if possible. So there was an issue about getting a translator involved and there was also an issue about acknowledging the different religious perspectives of these two personas. Whenever we meet there is always a discussion about how we deal with these things. Additionally, she is quite resistant to medication. That is, to the idea of medication; she's not resistant to medication when it is prescribed.

When showing her respect I'm aware there is a higher level of respect for older people in Asian communities than in the broader population. I needed to get her on side in order to accept that the medicine that I'm suggesting is appropriate. I couldn't break trust by forcing her to use a translator but still needed to make sure she understood why I was proposing she takes pills.

She understood about her schizophrenia in one sense, she had her model of it, though I'm not sure it was the medical model. She understood we were trying to give her medication to help her keep this invader at bay, but when, for example, she had side effects, she thought the very shaky hands came from the other woman inside her. Trying to explain that the tablets I was giving her for what I felt was a drug side effect might get rid of the effect of the woman inside her – trying to use her beliefs, not in the sense of sharing her delusion but in the sense of trying to tailor it to her beliefs was not easy. I don't think I ever fully achieved it, but it did open my eyes to the difficulties one has talking the same language with somebody, not just in terms of patients with linguistic differences. It's a problem I have with some native English speakers.

Inevitably the relationship developed. It wasn't a single consultation. Over time I learned ways of trying to accept that she was trying to speak my language while making it clear to her that though I couldn't speak her language I really wanted to understand what was happening to her so that I could make life a little better. It was about trying to make it very much about her and not much about me. My measure of success was her agreement to take the medication and in this case some external feedback on how she was getting on from the home she lived in.

For me this case reinforces the need to ensure that what I say is understood across the range of patients not just with those from other language backgrounds. She was difficult but likeable. Her model of the world was very different from mine. My perception didn't always match up with hers. Yet you felt that you had to keep helping – there was something about her. She lived in sheltered accommodation, so she was getting some help, but she was becoming more isolated even within that. She had physical problems as well, and there were issues about how she managed those.

She certainly broadened my view about what respecting someone is about. It was about trying to live in her world. This case brought the 'lifeworld' very much to the forefront of my thinking.

Dealing with Uncertainty

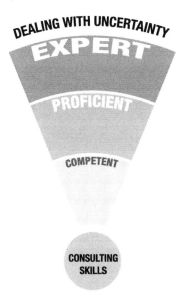

Figure 2.17 Dealing with Uncertainty – domain segment

Dealing with Uncertainty involves multi-tasking, since the doctor is not only making a clinical judgement but simultaneously assessing the soundness of that judgement, as well as looking at how much it would matter if s/he were wrong. Sometimes, against the odds, the unlikely happens. Every clinical judgement should therefore include a risk analysis. If this diagnosis turns out to be wrong, what are the possible alternatives and how dangerous are they? If there is danger, how much should we do to try to eliminate the possibility or deal with the danger when it comes? Do we refine the diagnosis or build a safety net into the management?

At expert level, this process should not only be shared with the patient, but the negotiation of how much risk to tolerate and how to manage it becomes a management tool in itself. The idea of concordance is implicit in this domain. However, achieving concordance can be difficult because of the inequality of the negotiation; the patient has the greater investment in safety, but the doctor has greater knowledge and the responsibility for the resources used. The negotiation should be productive diagnostically in revealing where the patient's anxieties lie and how the uncertainty impinges on his or her beliefs and values. It can be productive therapeutically, giving patients responsibility and making them active protagonists in their own welfare.

DEALING WITH UNCERTAINTY – WHAT IS KNOWN

- All clinical judgements are based on likelihoods, not certainties.

  'Uncertainty is ". . . a state of decision making in a probabilistic environment".'[38]

- The work of primary care is grounded in increasing (clinical) uncertainty.

  'The more an illness is studied within the context of a patient's life as a whole, the less reliable the standard explanations become.'[39]

  'The new flows of knowledge produced by IT systems, the effect of market forces on professional jurisdictions and the role of expertise in innovation all constitute a challenge to professional orthodoxy.'[40]

- Uncertainty is related to risk and its management.
- Uncertainty can be shared with the patient as part of management planning.

I was called on a home visit to see a lady 63 years old who two weeks previously had a hip replacement done. She was complaining of some pain in the leg so I went to see her because I was concerned (when you get a history like that you think of a DVT straight off). She was up and about on a frame and she said she had some pain in the leg but mainly at night. She mentioned particularly that the leg, although it was swollen, had been going down. I examined her. The leg was a bit swollen but no more than I expected for two weeks post op. It was a bit tender. It was not inflamed or reddened. On palpating it was a bit tender but not particularly so. At the end of examining her, at the back of my mind I still thought it could be a DVT but on balance I thought it wasn't. I discussed this with her and she said she wanted to be sure that it wasn't, and so we agreed that I would arrange for her to have a blood test. I had to do it the next day because I had missed the blood testing for that day. The next day I got the D-dimers result back in the late afternoon, which turned out to be 7000 and therefore I had to visit her with a view to admitting her to hospital.

- The ability to work with uncertainty depends upon the personal attributes and understanding of the doctor.

  'It took me some time in practice to realize that a fundamental aspect of family medicine was its attitude to uncertainty. After literally tens of thousands of consultations with patients, and many hundreds of house-calls, clinical practice eventually taught me one big, rather sobering lesson: it's the more you know about doctoring and why it works (or doesn't work), the more you realize how much you don't know.'[41]

> ## IN DEALING WITH UNCERTAINTY, CONSIDER:
>
> Context – situational understanding
> Communication – using a range of interpersonal skills
> Connectedness – 'going there'
> Completeness – holistic cover

- Patient-centred approaches increase the level of uncertainty.

  '. . . conflict between medical authority and patient autonomy is fundamental to the doctor-patient relationship . . .'[42]

  'Robust scientific conclusions are too sparse to inform fully most of the choices that physicians must make about tests and treatments. Instead ad hoc rules of thumb, or "heuristics" must guide them, and many of these are problematic.'[43]

DEALING WITH UNCERTAINTY – IN MY EXPERIENCE

CASE 1

The patient I am thinking about must be 20 now. She has been with the practice on and off for about four years, some of which time she has been in prison. We have immense problems because she is recurrently severely anaemic with a haemoglobin level of 7 and completely non-adherent with investigations, medication or hospital out-patient departments. The complicating factor at the moment is that she has a young child who is 45 weeks old. He came a month ago with a three-week history of diarrhoea and vomiting. At examination the child was completely normal – a happy child, well hydrated, doing all the right sort of things. She was given the usual advice and health visitor support.

She came back yesterday because the child was 'doing her head in' – keeping her up all night. He couldn't go and stay with grandma because the child screamed all night if he couldn't be with mum. She said he had stopped vomiting for four days but was now vomiting again, again and again. He'd seen the health visitor and been weighed. She hadn't got the Red Book (a patient-held child health record). She was back in 20 minutes saying she couldn't find the Red Book. During this time I managed to talk to the community health visitor. We both feel that this is a woman who is not coping and getting very close to child risk. The child's completely normal, happy and appears to be thriving but we don't have other weights to go on at the minute. Not pyrexial, not dehydrated, happy to be examined, no bruises, no rash. We can't get to the bottom of it.

She said, 'I went to the health visitor – useless'. She told the health visitor she didn't think much of us. The stories change. When she left me she went happily. If my child had been vomiting for six weeks I would be yelling. She is presenting cries for help and we have to find ways of dealing with that. She is to see the health visitor again tomorrow. She is going to try and find the Red Book and she is coming to see me next week.

The temptation was to give her a therapeutic trip down to see the paediatricians but I don't believe there is anything wrong with him.

Comment – In any complex case there will be uncertainty. It is worth contemplating how an inexperienced doctor might reconfigure a complex case of this kind into a complicated one that is capable of being solved. Notice how this doctor contained the uncertainty and did not attempt to 'solve' problems at this stage.

CASE 2

This was a woman my registrar had mentioned previously, but this time she said she couldn't cope and asked me to deal with it. The woman, in her twenties, was clearly very distressed, in a crumpled heap supported by her boyfriend.

The story was that she had been doing a degree in psychology, part of which had involved discussing some very disgusting crimes, including cannibalism. She had become fixated on these cases and started to find that she couldn't stop thinking about them, including child murder etc. She began to think that she may be going to commit these crimes – that she may be a Peter Sutcliffe in the making. She was very distressed – the more she tried to argue with herself that this wasn't the case the more she became fixated on the crimes. So she was terrified that she was a serious criminal in the making.

My registrar didn't have sufficient certainty to put her mind at rest. Whilst I also had a little bit of uncertainty, I was reassured by the quite warm character of the woman once I started speaking with her. So I decided that I would be assertive in reassuring her that this was in no way an indication of criminal propensity and that it wasn't a problem and all we needed to concentrate on was getting her mind away from the nasty fixations. With that very confident presentation she quickly calmed down and was able to accept some very practical means of focusing her mind on other areas of thought so she could stop ruminating. She left quite happily with a view to coming back in a short time.

Comment – The uncertainty was managed in this case by coming across to her with a certainty reassured by the incongruence in what she was proposing to do and her warm character.

Use of Resources

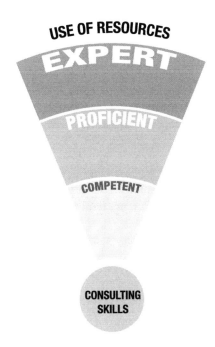

Figure 2.18 Use of Resources – domain segment

Risk may be reduced by throwing resources at an area of uncertainty until the need for judgement almost disappears. An expert avoids this profligacy by tightly defining those areas where need is unequivocal or risk is intolerable and allocating resources to them appropriately. Resources should also be used effectively: supporting evidence-based management of the correct target population. But the management must also be acceptable to the patient, to their values, ideas, beliefs and receptiveness, otherwise valuable resources may be wasted and the patient left unsatisfied. The expert doctor therefore ensures that the risk/effectiveness analysis is fully shared with the patient.

These disparate factors must also be put alongside the doctor's responsibility to the practice population as a whole in husbanding limited resources. The combination makes for complex judgements involving prioritisation of problems and plans.

USE OF RESOURCES – WHAT IS KNOWN

Use of Resources involves how *time* and how *resources* are utilised.

Use of time
- Priorities for the allocation of time will depend not only upon the presenting problem but upon the context in which the doctor is working – external time pressures and conflicting commitments as well as the physical environment.
- The doctor's agenda will develop with experience; the way in which a doctor frames a problem evolves through reflective and metacognitive processes.
- Time for effective and efficient negotiation with the patient is necessary.
- Negotiation will involve allowance of risk and the sharing of uncertainty, which is dependent upon an extended range of interpersonal skills.

Use of resources
- Tension exists between the drive for monetary value and quality.

I recently had a 35-year-old man who had developed low back pain and had previously seen other colleagues. The pain had become worse, with radiation down his leg. When I saw him he was in a lot of pain, causing him to limp. Clinically I had no doubt that he had a prolapsed intervertebral disc and there were some neurological signs to support this. I was a little worried because he had some vague urinary symptoms. He had some hesitancy and was going more frequently but there was no incontinence. On examination he had normal anal tone. I was a little concerned that he was getting worse and that it could lead to cauda-equina syndrome. I contacted the orthopaedic doctor on call, who felt that the patient's symptoms were not enough to require admission. But the problem needed to be sorted out fairly quickly. I discussed the case with the consultant radiologist and we agreed that an MRI scan would be done urgently. I felt this was the best option, as referring him to a clinic would have meant further delay. The patient was pleased the investigation was to be done in the very near future. Managing things in this manner involved significant cost to the practice, whereas if he had been referred the cost would have been defrayed to secondary care, but I felt this was justified in view of the clinical picture.

- It is desirable to have access to a comprehensive range of high-quality services, but with limited resources, efficiency, equity and quality of care are not always achievable. The patient will have a view on this.

  'Some problematic situations are situations of conflict among values. Medical technologies such as kidney dialysis or tomography have created demands that stretch the nation's willingness to invest in medical services. How should physicians respond to the conflicting requirements of efficiency, equity and quality of care?'[44]

- The doctor's degree of comfort in his or her surgery will result from the balance between personal values, patient needs, practice protocols and other environmental demands. There may be tensions between actions directed towards meeting QOF performance targets and patient-centred medicine; for example, some patients with elevated blood pressure do not wish to take allopathic medication.

I began consulting with a 20-year-old patient by asking him how the weekend had been. He had been seen by one of my colleagues three days before with suicidal ideation, and I noted he had been on antidepressants previously with little response. He talked about his music gig, the friends he had seen and the church he had visited. We talked about how much better he seemed. I allowed him to talk and discover for himself that there were strategies he could employ to lift his mood when at times he felt he was sinking. This seemed to strike a chord with him, and he reflected back that the other doctors 'were always trying to give me something from their box of tricks', which was not what he particularly wanted – he knew he had to get through this by himself and with his own resources.

USE OF RESOURCES – IN MY EXPERIENCE

CASE 1

A patient came to see me who, over the past five to seven years, has had increasing problems with apparent allergic reactions to a variety of stimuli. These episodes have increasingly resulted in her landing up in hospital and having various resuscitation efforts made. She is documented in the hospital as having a post-operative respiratory arrest, and in her most recent episode she was apparently heading towards respiratory arrest and so was resuscitated, including IV injection of adrenalin. The reason I discussed this with her at some length was that I'd had a phone call and a letter from one of the hospital specialists. He'd reviewed her records, having been called to see her following the latest episode, and felt strongly that she didn't have physical symptoms as such – he felt this was a serious case of conversion disorder.

The key was to spend time listening to her talking about the episodes and feeding back various parts of the story to her, showing different angles – how different people would have perceived it. One of her responses was 'so I am being over-medically managed'. She has previously had an issue with this along the line of 'should I be making complaints?' I explained that, 'No, because the physical picture she is presenting to the staff is one heading towards arrest of some form or another.' So it was a fairly heavy-going consultation in terms of actually getting her to listen.

Thinking back, I was silent a lot. I allowed her time to reflect on what I had said and to come back to me with different responses. I summarised what had been said to me and what had been written in the hospital letter. Explaining it in simple terms rather than going into medical terminology was crucial, i.e. the hospital doctor talked in terms of a serious conversion disorder – that there were real physical symptoms which were linked to her mental state rather than a true allergic response. There were various times when she got upset during the consultation.

This is potentially very grim news – from her perspective she does have real physical problems. She said, 'You are telling me that I am mad.' 'No, I am telling you that it is a slightly more complicated picture than a purely allergic problem.' If I see her in a couple of weeks, I'll find out whether she has blocked this information as she has done in the past after talk of pseudo-seizures. In the past she has then gone to one of the partners, so I said, 'You may choose not to see me after this conversation.' **Using time to contain her behaviour is important here so I'd already talked this through with the partners.**

CASE 2

Often a patient comes in and tells you about something very minor. I think of this particular chap who kept coming back to me and each time I knew there was something else he wasn't giving me. I tried everything I could and began to think, 'I'm rubbish, I know there's something else there. He's just not giving it to me.' I tried every clue until at the end of the day I thought, 'It's his consultation, yes, I know there is something he is not disclosing, but if he's not yet in a place where he will say it, then so be it.' I think there was initially a very inefficient use of resources because he kept coming back with things that clearly weren't the problem. Eventually he told me that it was impotence. It was just too much for him. When it did come out, I think we had done most of his preventative healthcare for the next 20 years. Sometimes you need to modify the resources employed until the patient is ready to use them.

Focus

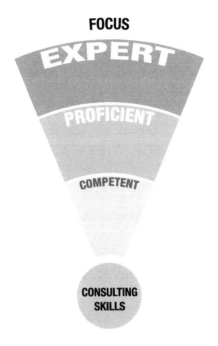

Figure 2.19 Focus – domain segment

This next domain reflects the extended ability of doctors to use (apparently) intuitive judgement. Intuitive decision making frees attention, enabling many themes and agendas to be heard and acted upon simultaneously and viewed in the dimensions of varied time scales and environmental contexts.

The doctor must listen to the patient's complaint, while recognising any emotional subtext, watching for physical signs, remembering past and family history, and putting the current problems in the context of the patient's social environment and overall clinical picture. At the same time, doctors must be recalling medical theory and fact, assessing available resources and planning future management. The skills of successful multi-tasking of this degree are termed *Focus*. They allow the doctor to maintain congruity of purpose despite apparently divergent or conflicting influences from presented dialogue, observation, memory and prior knowledge. They enable the doctor to respond more appropriately to each factor because of the ability to experience it in the context of all the others.

Focus allows doctors to be more timely in their interventions; rather than producing instant responses to patient information, they can hold their response ready while undertaking other tasks until the patient has become suitably receptive.

FOCUS – WHAT IS KNOWN

- At one level, focus involves 'being there' for the patient.
- At another level, because family doctor consulting is complex, always a matter of balancing ever-changing variables, maintaining focus demands highly developed and often creative use of consulting skills.
- Where the focus lies at any moment in time depends upon 'situational awareness'.[45]

> **Situational awareness** – the perception of elements in the environment within a volume of time and space, the comprehension of their meaning, and the projection of their status in the near future.[46]
>
> For experienced practitioners, situational awareness is that instant, reflex mode of action – affected by time constraints – that will later be found to have been a response to:
> - who is in the room?
> - how are they feeling?
> - how are they relating?
> - what are they expecting?
> - where do I fit in here?
>
> Situational awareness functions like a radar. It develops through metacognitive attentiveness – the ability to suspend in time, from premature judgement, and in space, from what is before you – sometimes referred to as the 'helicopter view'. The ability to develop such an 'aerial' view develops over time.

I walked into the room. There was my patient (a French-speaking Congolese woman whose baby had died soon after birth), her friend, a translator and me. The patient, I knew, had a history of psychosis. I didn't know how things would go. It became apparent the friend and the translator were on the same positive wavelength so I began to relax.

- Focus is concerned with directing the flow of traffic on the 'bridge between teller and listener' together with the ability to hold and park issues.
- Focus involves the willingness to 'go there' (*see* p. 156). Going there is only possible if the doctor is 'present' (see below) in the consultation.

> Presence can be described as 'coupling with reality' or 'letting come'. It involves the ability to detach yourself and avoid predetermining outcomes – the ability to hold and utilise uncertainty in the consultation. Presence or 'being there' ensures as many ideas as possible are expressed and explored and that cues and clues are more likely to be picked up and responded to.[47]

I think of a lady who came in the other day; she was very proud that she had five problems. She elucidated those five problems. One, she wanted a medication review, two she was concerned about her blood pressure, three was her migraines, four was that she was getting some joint pains particularly in her feet, and I think the fifth may have been as simple as wanting a repeat prescription. She had five but they weren't five for me. Take the fifth, let's say it was a repeat prescription, well, that links to whatever else goes on in the consultation. I wouldn't call that a problem; it's a consultation outcome. For the medication review I needed to know that her blood pressure wasn't working for her, as her migraines may well not be migraines but, maybe, headaches related to the blood pressure. The text books say there aren't any but it's amazing how many patients you see where it does relate. And the problems in her feet were gout due to the diuretics she was on for her blood pressure. She outlined it as five things – it comes back to the problem-solving thing – for me five things aren't five things.

FOCUS – IN MY EXPERIENCE

I saw this lady in her seventies a couple of weeks ago. She was waiting on the landing, and I went out to collect her. She was there with her husband but he didn't come in. She came in and sat down slowly and gingerly. From the record it was evident that there was such a lot of medical history and drugs that I knew it was going to be a difficult consultation for a first time of meeting. She mentioned her initial problem: a swollen finger. It turned out she got swelling in her finger that she'd previously experienced as gout. She'd seen the nurse, who had cut off her wedding rings. That seemed a big deal to me but apparently less so to her. I thought it would be playing on her mind but she had a lot of other issues to discuss.

We discussed the gout and previous treatments and the pain she was still having. Alongside this were other issues; one was 'limey' urine, which caught me on the hop as I'd never heard of that before. That was the way she described the colour. She was querying whether she had an infection but she was not really worried – she didn't have any symptoms. The other thing she brought up was the fact that she was on warfarin, a major factor in how I managed her. She was due for an INR in a few days. We had a look through her warfarin book to see what her control was like – relatively stable.

She also went on to talk about pains in her shoulders, around the shoulder blade as well, which she thought was related to the finger. That was the initial couple of problems.

She went on to say that yesterday she had been very unwell with a fever, 'at death's door'. Another issue was her breathing. When she came in she was huffing and puffing and clearly overweight. From the records she had several problems with her breathing and previously had a blood clot in her lungs. I didn't know whether this breathing was normal for her or not. With so many problems already, my problem was, 'what can I leave out today?' I made a conscious decision not to take on the breathing. I went on to examine her fingers, temperature and feel of her tummy to make sure she had no signs of pyelonephritis or kidney infection, because she'd mentioned the temperature. The swelling around the finger was consistent with the gout.

I ran through the options for her, explaining that she was complicated. She understood that well enough. We discussed the gout and the urinary symptoms. She'd previous been treated for the gout – with colchicine. With the warfarin, we are struggling with any anti-inflammatories plus the fact that she is already on other medication. As I was writing the scripts she mentioned that she didn't want anything with 'e's (e numbers). Because I knew this consultation could be never-ending, I let this flow over me. Though I was listening intently, I was deliberately not responding. Despite having several previous episodes of gout and using the same treatment, I think she felt adequately treated. I arranged for her to have blood and urine tests, as she was coming back later in the week.

When I asked her whether she would take the colchicine, she said, 'I'm not thick you know.' We both smiled.

A few days later she saw her usual doctor, who referred her to a renal physician, as her blood and urine tests had come back as abnormal.

Synthesising Skills (responding flexibly)

The list of domains already described includes a formidable collection of skills. Intuitive, reflective, holistic, proactive and interactive consulting may lead to a wide range of complex judgements and priorities to be arrived at in any one consultation. Doctors may have immediate problems to be dealt with or may aspire to achieve longer-term goals with their patients. They may decide their patients are not yet sufficiently receptive for a particular line of management and that it must be delayed while groundwork is undertaken. They may realise that they are being the wrong sort of doctor for this patient at this particular time, and that they should modify their behaviour to be more immediately acceptable to their patients' expectations and benefit their short-term needs. Additionally, they may alter the doctor–patient dynamics to become more productive in the longer term.

Expert doctors will therefore be faced with a range of possible actions to be prioritised. They will need to make long- and short-term strategies regarding the

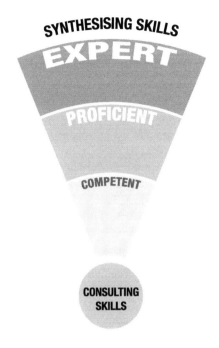

Figure 2.20 Synthesising Skills – domain segment

presenting agendas, the consultation transactions, the doctor–patient relationship, the future medical and social needs, the family and employment perspectives and the resource issues. The ability to take an overview of all these aspects of their patients' needs during the process of consulting is fundamental to deliberate practice.[48] Combining this overview with the capacity to modify the deployment of available skills and resources to maximum effect is a domain of skills in itself.

SYNTHESISING SKILLS – WHAT IS KNOWN

> 'Synthesis – *the putting together of elements and parts so as to form a whole. This involves the process of working with pieces, parts, elements etc., and arranging and combining them in such a way as to constitute a pattern or structure not clearly there before.'*[49]

- Synthesising Skills involve combining and integrating the competencies and skills of all the other domains to form a unique whole – unique in the sense that the synthesising does not represent a proposed set of operations or specifications to be carried out but is reflective of the uniqueness of the individuals concerned.

'Scientific reasoning is an exploratory dialogue that can always be resolved into two voices or two episodes of thought, imaginative and critical, alternate and interact. In the imaginative episode we form an opinion, take a view, make an informed guess, which might explain the phenomena under investigation. The generative effect is the formation of a hypothesis.' [50]

'Evidence based medicine (EBM) is the integration of research evidence with clinical expertise and patient values. When these three elements are integrated, clinicians and patients form a diagnostic and therapeutic alliance which optimizes clinical outcomes and quality of life.' [51]

- Synthesis of skills results in a 'generative' effect whereby the outcome of the whole is greater than the summation of the outcomes of the individual parts. The resultant generative effect reflects the need for holistic approaches and a mutual respect for the individuality of the patient and doctor concerned. Choice, flexibility and adaptability are key markers of Synthesising Skills.

  'The process by which we formulate a hypothesis is not logical but non logical, i.e. outside logic.' [52]

- Synthesis involves attempting to derive abstract relations from a detailed analysis. The relations are not explicit from the outset – they have to be discovered or deduced.

  '. . . a story which we invent and criticise and modify as we go along, so that it ends by being, as nearly as we can make it, a story about real life.' [53]

- Concordant consultation outcomes indicate an act of synthesis.

DOCTORS' WORK – OR WHY SYNTHESISING SKILLS ARE NECESSARY

Doctors' work routinely presents them with problems for analysis, solutions, and advice which are complex and multifaceted, requiring knowledge and skills extending from bioscience through statistics and behavioural science to counselling. These problems are frequently multidimensional and not amenable to simple algorithmic solutions. These require case-specific investigations to permit their nature to be properly defined and understood. Medicine's content and its practices are broad and ill defined, and subject to constant updating by a large research literature, requiring continuing, lifelong understanding of the research mentality and the changing theories

> it produces. **Challenges and problems are thus encountered for which standard solutions are not available and for which novel resolutions will routinely be needed,** requiring the developed understanding of risk and probability, and highly sophisticated judgements based on experience and embedded in the live academic literature and professional practice.[54]

SYNTHESISING SKILLS – IN MY EXPERIENCE

This was a woman in her early thirties who came complaining of tiredness, but once she sat down she admitted it was due to stress. It turned out that she had a boyfriend who she was very fond of. He'd had a chequered past with alcohol problems. She was living with him and it turned out that he had massive debts that he had ignored for many years and she was having to support him to the tune of £35 000 – all her savings really – to bail him out. What worried her was that he was a man who ran away from problems and she was concerned that he was still drinking.

She obviously had great affection for this person. She talked very warmly about him and the hard time he had had in the past and how much affection he could give her, but she was obviously very hurt by what he was doing and the risk she was having to take. I felt that she needed some sort of reassurance that she could take a firm line. So I made a conscious decision to stop counselling and go into a paternalistic role. I told her that if he wanted her and was worthy of her and he was prepared to accept all that money from her, she should expect that he should make a serious effort to do something about the drinking and that she should tell him so. She was very pleased with that reassurance and went out looking much happier. I was a little bit nervous that I had given her very direct advice, which is something I don't normally do in that didactic way. A few days later I happened to see the boyfriend, who told me that he'd had a serious talk with his girlfriend and that it had cleared the air – she was a lot happier and he was making serious efforts to put his drinking right. I feel that the gamble I took paid off in the end.

> *'When time is extremely short, decisions have to be rapid and the scope for reflection is extremely limited. In those circumstances, reflection is best seen as a metacognitive process in which the practitioner is alerted to the problem, rapidly reads the situation, decides what to do and proceeds in a state of continuing alertness.'*[55]

WHAT WE MEAN BY – PERFORMANCE LEVELS

Initially, the Consultation Expertise Model was developed for two reasons:

i. to help experienced practitioners critically reflect on their consulting practice

ii. to provide trainees and new family doctors with aspirational targets for developing their consulting performance.

The many excellent and rigorous frameworks for assessing consulting performance in terms of basic skills and competencies of necessity focus on minimal requirements. For example, any assessment leading to certification for independent family medicine, such as the Observation of Consulting component of the nMRCGP,[56] looks at the competencies which every family doctor must have by the beginning of their career. We wanted something that was relevant to us as hardened professionals that we could use repeatedly to demonstrate that we were at the top of our game, not that we were above the bottom. The framework we required would need to specifically address the issue of experience and have a number of stages within it. Each stage would need to have some degree of distinction from the adjacent stage in the sequence, but as we were not interested in being able to rank our performance there was no need for each stage to be discrete: stages could overlap or even share features. The whole point of the exercise was to use critical reflection to inform where we were in the sequence of stages so that we could improve our practice. The model required should be developmental. Most importantly, **it should specifically include elements that would be representative of expertise to guide the direction of learning**.

You will have guessed that we could not find anything suitable in the medical literature. Then one of us came across the writings of the Dreyfus brothers. Hubert is a philosopher and Stuart a mathematician who also plays chess. Together they had become interested in expert systems, essentially computer programs whose writers claimed could develop to take over human thinking – or in one case walking. To the Dreyfus brothers it seemed questionable whether a computer could ever replicate the processes of the human mind, so they set out to work out how the human expert mind worked. They could then demonstrate differences between expert practice and rule-based machine working. So they talked to pilots, managers and chess players and developed a five-stage sequential framework leading to expert practice. The full story of what they concluded can be read in *Mind over Machine*.[57] Here, though, is a summary framework of the Dreyfus's model as developed by Michael Eraut:

SUMMARY OF DREYFUS MODEL OF SKILL ACQUISITION[58]

Level 1: Novice
Rigid adherence to taught rules or plans.
Little situational perception.
No discretionary judgement.

Level 2: Advanced Beginner
Guidelines for action based on attributes or aspects, i.e. aspects are characteristics of situations recognisable only after some prior experience.
Situational perception still limited.
All attributes and aspects are treated separately and given equal importance.

Level 3: Competent
Coping with crowdedness.
Now sees actions at least partially in terms of longer-term goals.
Conscious of deliberate planning.
Standardised and routinised procedures.

Level 4: Proficient
Sees situations holistically rather than in terms of aspects.
Sees what is most important in a situation.
Perceives deviations from the normal pattern.
Decision making less laboured.
Uses maxims for guidance, whose meaning varies according to the situation.

Level 5: Expert
No longer relies on rules, guidelines or maxims.
Intuitive grasp of situations based on deep tacit understanding.
Analytical approaches used only in novel situations or when problems occur.
Vision of what is possible.

The first important point is that this classification is **context specific**. You wouldn't want a grand master at chess flying you to Barcelona would you?

So which context are we interested in? We agreed that it is the clinical encounter with a patient in the family medicine consulting room. As professionals we have to be assessed as competent, so for convenience we agreed that we would overlap the Dreyfus 'competent' with competence as assessed for certification in family medicine, but please note that this is only for convenience and to avoid confusion. The Dreyfus category of 'competent' describes a pattern of mental activities that apply to any form of clinical or other practice: successful completion of nMRCGP defines us as being competent to perform all the tasks of family medicine in the UK.[59]

We have mapped the five stages onto a family doctor career like this:

NOVICE	ADVANCED BEGINNER	COMPETENT	PROFICIENT	EXPERT
Pre-clinical	Clinical student Doctors 1–5 years after qualifying	Certified family doctor	Family doctor – maybe with five years' practice	Family doctor – possibly thereafter

You will have noticed immediately that movement across the categories is related to experience. At the novice/advanced beginner stage, knowledge development is important, but expertise is dependent upon relevant experience in the practice context, i.e. consulting with patients. This sometimes causes confusion. In our experience, family doctors in training sometimes describe a colleague as 'expert' because they see behaviour that impresses them. A family doctor trainee **cannot** be expert by virtue of lacking relevant experience. On the other hand, there may be doctors with adequate experience who do not become expert. This comes about from the way that such doctors process experience. (Remember the joke about there being fools and experienced fools?) In fact, in the Dreyfus model, the transition from one stage to another represents a change in our way of thinking. As a consequence, there has to be a change in our learning to maintain progression.

A **novice** needs to develop basic knowledge: facts, facts, facts. This is how to take a history, these are the features of tonsillitis, and eye contact helps communication. But these facts are context-free. They can be known and learned without any form of consulting practice. It's just a question of following the **rules**.

Advanced beginners learn how to apply the rules in the context of practice situations. Each encounter with, say, a patient with a sore throat leads to a comparison with previous similar situations. The learning is about which rules to apply under which circumstances. The learning is similar to following **guidelines** (when this happens, do this). No wonder experienced doctors can have difficulty when they are given guidelines to follow.

By the time doctors have qualified and completed training for family medicine, they have a huge range but not depth of experience. Many of these experiences are similar or overlap. When they do, it becomes possible to recognise a **pattern** from only a few pieces of the full picture. It is not necessary to take a full history or to examine the whole respiratory system to know that this is a self-limiting viral infection. Under pressure, it is important to decide which bits of the full picture are needed to be sure enough of the pattern. There is no time to obtain too much detail or certainty. To be a **competent** doctor (in the Dreyfus sense), the learning needs to be about actions that are important for the longer-term aims and goals of practice: in this case, ensuring that all those who need to consult have the opportunity to do so.

Our interest, though, lies in the concept of expertise; beyond this point in the progression it becomes more and more difficult to talk with meaning without including the context of the practice being talked about. A context-free description doesn't make sense or is ambiguous. If I tell you that a feature of expert practice is **fluency**, you may be uncertain as to what I mean. If I ask a trainee to recall an episode when they watched their trainer deal smoothly and easily with a difficult issue that they would have found impossible without having pauses in the conversation for thought and reflection, they would probably know what I am referring to. When we are working with patient simulations, the simulators often tell us that they can tell trainers from family doctor trainees: trainees need to stop and think; the consultation moves in fits and starts as they think their way through the consultation; consulting with trainers flows like a conversation. This is what fluency is about. When watching a fluent consultation things just seem to happen. We may also be surprised that apparently significant information appears to be discarded or ignored without being considered.

Fluent practice in consulting may be described as **intuitive**, and it is important to be clear what is meant by this. If an intuitive consulter is asked to describe what they were doing during the consultation, they are likely to refer to previous experiences of patients who many times presented with similar patterns of illness and degrees of severity. Fluency develops when the consulter recognises a pattern and repeats effective action from a previous experience. Experience of effective intervention has led to 'know-how'. Intuitive or fluent consulting is the application of 'know-how' without the need for continual deliberation – '*competent performance is rational; proficiency is transitional and experts act arationally*'.[60] Intuition is not the application of some mystical and indefinable process but grows out of experience of successful practice.

Fluency is driven by 'know-how'.

'We shall use "intuition" and "know how" as synonymous.'[61]

Both **proficient** and **expert** consulting requires 'know-how' or intuitive responses during the consultation. The difference lies in the response to the intuition. A proficient consulter will still need to analyse what to do following the intuition. So thinking of a patient with a sore throat, as we begin to talk about self-care we may notice that the patient becomes more assertive, and intuitively we recognise a pathway that leads to dispute about the need for antibiotics. If we are proficient we will need to scan consciously our repertoire of approaches to decide what to do next. An expert will change tack intuitively without perhaps even noticing that they have adjusted their approach.

We should not expect, however, that an expert will do everything intuitively. When things run smoothly there is no problem. To quote Dreyfus:

> *'When things are going normally, experts don't solve problems and don't make decisions; they do what normally works.'*[62]

Note the 'normally'. Family medicine is full of the unexpected and non-normal. Sometimes things that worked well in the past just won't work this time. Then the expert will stop and reflect critically on their intuition before proceeding.

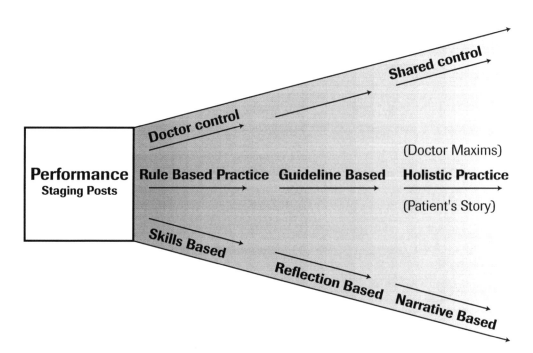

Figure 2.21 Performance staging posts

WHAT WE MEAN BY – INDICATIVE STATEMENTS

Now might be a good moment to take stock of how our understanding of the Model is developing.

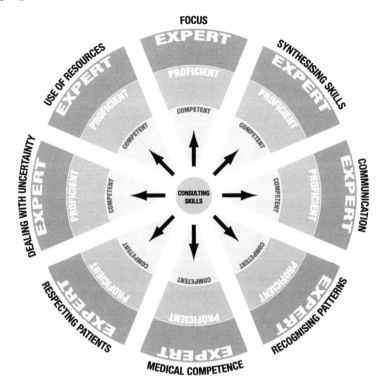

Figure 2.22 The Model so far – consulting skills + domains + performance levels

We began by trying to understand what we meant by the concept of 'expertise'. This led us to describe a number of **domains,** each one of which is a necessary but insufficient component of expertise. Domains may be difficult to distinguish clearly from one another or they may overlap. This does not matter, as their primary purpose is to help develop our understanding. We can describe a domain, but we may not be able to define it. We know when we are in the territory of the domain, but it is harder for us to say when we are leaving that territory for another domain. Urban environments are familiar to us all, but it is difficult to describe at what point we enter suburbia. At many times there will be elements of both urban and suburban environments present together. The nMRCGP curriculum is also written with reference to domains, which are explained in Core Statement – Being a GP.[63]

Within each domain of expertise, we introduced three **performance levels**: competent, proficient and expert. The nMRCGP also recognises three performance levels: 'not yet competent', 'competent' and 'excellent' – excellence being defined in relation to the standard of the nMRCGP examination. The terms are different because the purpose of the nMRCGP examination is to demonstrate sufficient competence to be licensed as a family doctor.

You will remember that the starting point for our expertise work was to ask how we could help experienced practitioners develop an understanding of their professional work beyond repeated assessments of basic competence. To develop beyond 'competent', professional experience is an absolute requirement, so the performance levels in the Model have different titles from the performance levels of the nMRCGP.

Now we need to agree how we make judgements about which level of performance we are watching. In the early stages of development of the Model we found this difficult because with increasing experience doctors become able to integrate several competencies in an interaction with a patient. For example, a doctor may hear a cue that she would like to pursue but is hearing what she thinks is an important piece of psychological background information. She decides that it is a better use of time to allow the psychological background to evolve rather than to pursue the cue. At the same time she is holding the focus and judging whether there will be a further opportunity to consider the cue that has been presented without disturbing the flow of the consultation.

One way of assessing a consultation is to have a list of performance criteria against which to judge a doctor's performance. This is how assessments of consulting are made in the nMRCGP. Performance Criterion (PC) 2 states:

> *'The doctor is seen to respond to signals (cues) that lead to a deeper understanding of the problem.'*[64]

That criterion is appropriate for a family doctor specialist registrar at the end of training, but how would our experienced doctor perform against it? In the example above she might not be assessed as performing well at all. This is the same problem that experienced drivers have in taking the standard driving test. Not many of us move our heads to look in the rear-view mirror after we have been driving for some time. Does this mean that we are unaware of what is happening behind us?

When thinking about expertise, we have chosen not to use single performance criteria to determine the level of performance within a domain. We call the statements that we have chosen 'indicative'. **Indicative statements** help to describe what behaviours we would expect to see within each performance level, but they also set out how the behaviour is expected to change as we move from one performance level to another.

So let's return to our example of the experienced doctor apparently not responding to a cue. In the Communication domain we are prompted to consider whether a doctor 'responds to and uses cues in a seamless manner'. If we don't think this is so we need to consider the equivalent statement in the next performance level down and decide whether she 'identifies verbal and non-verbal cues'.

You will notice that there is an opportunity for us to recognise that the doctor has not responded immediately to a cue and has waited for an opportunity to respond later in the consultation so as not to disrupt the flow of the conversation. Other examples of how the indicative statements are used to form a judgement can be found in the fingerprint analysis of three doctors' consultations with Mrs Margaret Henderson that follows.

Notice the importance of the way we gather evidence: we are interested in looking for evidence of expertise **first.** Only if we do not find it do we look elsewhere to judge how to assess the doctor's performance. We are not interested in demonstrating that the doctor is competent. That has already been decided and we assume it. Nor are we interested in finding faults with the doctor's behaviour. We are interested in building up a picture of a doctor who has developed expertise through experience, a doctor who has learned to synthesise a number of competencies over time and apply them for the patient's benefit. We therefore look only for **positive evidence** of expert behaviour.

Each domain has a number of indicative statements. In some domains – see for example, Dealing with Uncertainty – there are more indicative statements at higher performance levels. Some indicative statements clearly relate to the nMRCGP performance indicators, but others do not. In all cases notice how the language of the indicative statement changes at each performance level.

The number of indicative statements can create a difficulty. What do we do if a doctor shows evidence of expertise in relation to some of the indicative statements but not in others? We have found that in this situation it helps to remember that we are collecting positive evidence of expertise. If there is clear evidence of some expert behaviour, then we are saying that this doctor is more than proficient. To be expert does not require expertise to be shown in all areas of a domain in all consultations at all times. Use of the indicative statements can be likened to pond dipping as illustrated in Figure 2.23.

USING INDICATIVE STATEMENTS – AN ILLUSTRATIVE CASE

The case of simulated patient Margaret Henderson, as seen by three doctors at different experience levels, will be used alongside the indicative statements for each domain to show how a consultation might be marked.

Case example – Margaret Henderson

Mrs Margaret Henderson, a 49-year-old computer operator in the NHS, presents with backache. She enters the consulting room looking physically tense, with a pale, resigned demeanour. Consulting doctors are provided with the following details:

Patient Number: 1526	
Sex	F
Surname	Henderson
Forename	Margaret
Date of Birth	49 yrs
Title	Mrs
Marital Status	Married
Medical Record Problems	
Significant Problems	
10 yr ago	TAH BSO – HRT Oestradiol implant
12 yr ago	Childbirth (M)
14 yr ago	Childbirth (M)
Surgery Entries	
2 m ago	HRT implant review BP 130/80
2 m ago	Letter from Chest Clinic –start new medication
3 m ago	Seen in Chest Clinic – COPD
6 m ago	SOB lung function tests consistent with COPD. Refer to Chest Clinic
9 m ago	Chest infection Rx erythromycin
10 m ago	Chest infection Rx cephalexin. Given up smoking
12 m ago	Chest infection Rx erythromycin. Smokes 40/day
Values	
10 m ago	Given up smoking
12 m ago	Smokes 40/day
Referrals	
6 m ago	Refer to Chest Clinic – COPD

Medication	
Current Date Commenced	Drug Detail
2 m ago	QVAR 100 2D Spiriva 15 mg daily Ipratroprium inhaler prn meloxicam 7.5 mg bd Co-codamol 8/500 prn

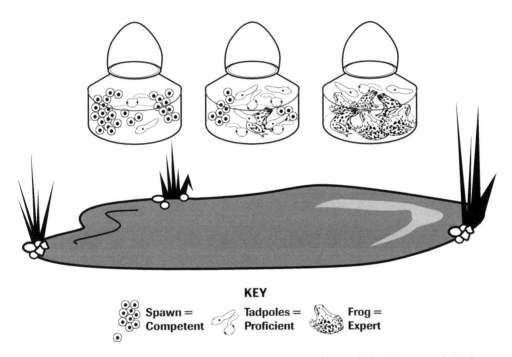

KEY

Spawn = Competent   Tadpoles = Proficient   Frog = Expert

Figure 2.23 Using indicative statements to determine expertise levels is akin to pond dipping

Mrs Henderson was filmed consulting with 20 doctors in their own surgeries over a period of weeks. All concerned were familiar with the protocols of simulated patient consulting – treat the patient as a real patient, and if and when examination is required say 'I'd like to examine you', and the patient will either consent to be examined or provide a card with the examination results. In this case the simulator had been taught how to respond on examination, so a near-reality situation was possible.

Doctors were asked to 'consult in your own way in a context where there are no exceptional time pressures.'

Word-for-word transcripts made from three consultations illustrate a variety of interactions with the same patient. A member of the project team subsequently analysed the transcripts using the indicative statements to provide a description and fingerprint.

Summary narratives – three doctors consult with Mrs Henderson
The following analytical narratives were made from observation of the recorded consultations:

Doctor 1
There are three equal parts to the consultation sequence. History-taking explores the nature and context of the back pain and medication, impinging on the patient's lifeworld briefly to establish the extent to which the back pain affects everyday life. A full examination is followed by non-probing questions regarding life stresses and mood. Two lifeworld cues, 'much to my husband's disgust I've got a cleaner' and 'Yes, I used to do that but recently – one thing and another', are not followed up.

Chronic obstructive pulmonary disease (COPD), though mentioned as a contributory problem by the patient, is not brought into the consultation. The patient discloses that she does not like taking tablets and feels she needs something such as injections or an epidural. Deeper concerns are not elicited. The doctor discusses injection and epidural and proposes that a combination of painkillers, exercise and physiotherapy would be helpful. The management third of the consultation is concerned with information – suggestion and negotiation around the doctor's proposal for action.

Interpersonal interaction is dominated by open, closed and echo questions, followed by suggestion and information around acceptance of the doctor's proposals. The consultation is kept within the bounds of the medical agenda, i.e. the problem as presented at progression level one.

Doctor 2
The consultation follows a three-stage sequence of medical-social history-taking (seven minutes), examination during which more socio-psychological information is disclosed (nine minutes) and a management discussion (five minutes) of alternative therapies, medication possibilities and physiotherapy (the local physiotherapist offers acupuncture). Orthopaedic surgery is mentioned but not considered appropriate (discussion of bulging disc on sciatic nerve). The patient is asked to consider various options, having come with the notion of injections or an epidural.

The question of stress-related home factors and the additional restriction of COPD are considered. An offer is made to talk about the matrimonial relationship problems at another time.

The outcome is referral to orthopaedic surgeons for assessment and a prescription issued on the basis of paracetamol for normal pain control and codeine for the really bad times.

Interpersonal skills in use are closed, open, circular and probing questions, nods, 'ums', 'ahs', empathy, signposting, clarification, informing and summary. The head-shaking response to, 'And how are things going, having a lot of pain can create stress at home', is followed up.

Doctor 3

This consultation takes the longest time of all three. The doctor listens to what the patient has to say about the back pain and asks for clarification as to how this has affected home and work life. She then puts this into a clinical context by asking about the outcomes of hospital visits and checks what investigations have been made. She then returns to the issue of how the back is affecting home and work and agrees with the patient that some form of extra help is needed. At this stage it is not determined what this help should be. Only now does she examine the back. During the examination she asks a few closed questions to exclude serious illness.

Following the examination she thinks aloud to the patient about how they could 'move things forward', and they agree together that the key problem affecting home and work is 'mobility'. They agree on a management plan.

The doctor allows a discussion about the marriage relationship to develop, even though it appears clear what she considers the next step to be. She talks with the patient about the experience of chronic illness and that some people need personal support for this. When it is clear that this is not forthcoming from the marriage, she signposts that support services are available but does not refer directly, leaving the patient room to consider this option.

She acknowledges the complexity of the patient's problem and suggests that they start 'somewhere' to begin to try to 'change things'. Having received confirmation from the patient that this 'feels like a step forward', she reviews and summarises the management plan.

Communication – Mrs Henderson case responses

Doctor 1

Doctor 1 signals early on his medical approach:

Doctor: *What's the problem?* before asking a series of clinically appropriate closed questions, some of which he accepts without elaboration: *'Are you working at the moment?'*

COMMUNICATION

EXPERT
- Encourages patient to respond.
- Employs reflective clarification, e.g. summarising.
- Responds to and uses verbal and non-verbal cues in a seamless manner.
- Uses language in a patient-centred manner.
- Tests mutual understanding.
- Assimilates social differences and cultures into management plan.

PROFICIENT
- Allows patient to elaborate.
- Clarifies details further.
- Identifies verbal and non-verbal cues.
- Uses language appropriately.
- Checks patient's understanding of doctor's intention.
- Responds to social differences and cultures.

COMPETENT
- Accepts things at face value.
- Picks up obvious verbal cues.
- Uses clear and simple language.
- Does not always check understanding.
- Acknowledges social differences and cultures.

CONSULTING SKILLS

This category examines the communication skills (as defined in the core of the model) exhibited by the practitioner within a consultation. Central to this category is the doctor's response to cues.*

How to distinguish the different levels of performance

Expert
Communication is patient-centred rather than doctor-centred. Verbal and non-verbal cues are used to maximal effect and the patient's understanding is not only checked but confirmed with testing. The doctor utilises the art of summarising and also positively encourages the patient to respond. The final management plan is fully negotiated with the patient, and any social/cultural differences are incorporated both within the consultation and that plan.

Proficient
The doctor is able to identify both verbal and non-verbal cues and adapts to social and cultural differences. The doctor grades their language appropriately, and the patient is allowed greater active participation in the consultation.

Competent
This links into basic levels of communication such as recognising verbal cues and an acknowledgement of social/cultural differences.

When fingerprinting, look for:

- verbal and non-verbal cues from the patient to assess what is picked up and used by the doctor
- both the doctor and patient's tone of voice, verbal cues and body language
- whether any references to cultural/social differences are incorporated into the management plan

*cues = information, verbal or non-verbal, that must be addressed.

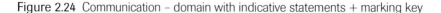

Communication relates to:
- Medical Competence – it enables the doctor to acquire the information necessary to make appropriate diagnoses.
- Dealing with Uncertainty – the doctor actions their diagnoses through negotiation with the patient. They must clearly and confidently communicate where uncertainty and risk lie.
- Respecting Patients – good communication enables the doctor to establish and develop their rapport with the patient.

Figure 2.24 Communication – domain with indicative statements + marking key

Patient:	*Um*
Doctor:	*What sort of job do you do?*
Patient:	*I'm a computer manager in the NHS.*
Doctor:	*Do you sit most of the day?*
Patient:	*Yes*
Doctor:	*How much are you active outside?* and so on.

This approach means that the doctor misses some clues when the patient talks about her husband: *'Much to my husband's disgust, I have got a cleaner'* but responds 'Oh that's good'. Later he asks, *'Have you any other stresses in your life?'*, to which the patient replies, *'Yes, like everybody else I suppose.'* The doctor doesn't respond to this but asks a specific question about low mood.

Doctor 2

Doctor 2 invites the patient to tell her story in her own way: *'I notice from your notes that you came . . . about a year and a half ago. So tell me a bit about what has been going on since then.'* The doctor does not ask a clinical question (*'Does anything get rid of that pain?'*) until the patient has been speaking for about two minutes.

The doctor then asks a series of questions and perhaps does not pick up on some clues:

Doctor:	*Do you work?*
Patient:	*Yes*
Doctor:	*What do you do?*
Patient:	*I work as a computer manager in the Health Service.*
Doctor:	*How's that going?*
Patient:	*Well, I do just carry on. I manage to work.*
Doctor:	*You've not had a lot of time off work?*
Patient:	*No. I get to work and that's sometimes a bit difficult actually getting to work but I go on with it and change my chair.*

Maybe a statement similar to the opening remark would have been helpful here: *'Tell me about the difficulties at work.'* It appears that the doctor has the necessary skills to allow the patient to tell a story but that at times they are not available to the doctor when needed. They have not become automatic or tacit.

The doctor is able to recognise and make use of non-verbal clues. While talking about the home situation the doctor asks, *'Having a lot of pain can create stress at home – how are things going?'* The patient says nothing but shakes her head. The doctor responds to this by saying, *'Not so good by the looks of it.'*

When discussing management plans, like Doctor 3 below, Doctor 2 talks of 'we' but in a slightly different way: *'We've tried you on painkillers'* and *'Now we've got a few choices available, things we can do for you now.'* The 'we' here seems to refer to doctors. Contrast this with the way an expert doctor uses 'we' to mean the doctor and the patient.

Doctor 3

From the beginning of the consultation, Doctor 3 flags that she is listening. She tells the patient that she has just had a *'quick flip through the notes to see what has been happening to you over the past few months'* and then invites her to *'tell me why you are here.'* She then allows the patient to do the majority of the talking. She does not ask a set of clinical questions in a sequence but follows the patient's story. When she talks about work she asks some clarifying questions (*'Have you made any adjustments at work to help you?'*). She chooses to introduce a discussion about other clinical problems: *'Now obviously the other main problem . . . is the chest you've got. That's obviously been giving you a bit of trouble over the last few months as well.'* Her language is personal (*'giving you a bit of trouble'*) rather than clinical. When the patient mentions she feels *'quite ashamed'* in relation to her smoking, she immediately asks her to clarify what she means: *'Why do you use the word ashamed?'*

The doctor is not afraid to 'go there' (*see* Going there, p.156).When the patient is telling her about her daily life, she remarks: *'Do you have anyone else you can share that with? You know, how you feel – two fairly chronic problems. Must get you down?'* The patient doesn't respond, so the doctor doesn't pursue it, but a few moments later when they are discussing drugs she checks her understanding again. When she comments: *'They've helped to a degree but not totally, otherwise I wouldn't be here. But you know it's the fact that . . .'* the doctor offers *'You are struggling?'*, and the patient agrees, *'Yes I am a bit.'*

When developing the management plan, the doctor uses inclusive language: *'I think **we** are going to have to start thinking about what **we** are going to have to do.'* When she does make suggestions, it is in a way that allows the patient to respond. Before suggesting the bone density scan, she introduces it like this: *'So I would have thought – I don't know how you think about this – there's a couple of ways forward.'* She checks the plan with the patient again, using personal language: *'So have we got an acceptable plan?'*, and then summarises it before the patient leaves.

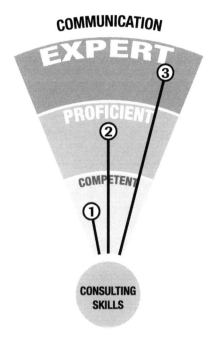

Figure 2.25 Communication – fingerprint markings

Recognising Patterns – Mrs Henderson case responses
Doctor 1
Doctor 1 establishes a detailed clinical picture based on his history and examination. The pattern he works with is exclusively medical, with no social dimension, even though he has asked some questions about life at home. Consequently, when he and the patient come to discussing treatment options he has nothing new to offer, as the patient has tried everything in the medical pattern already.

Doctor 2
Doctor 2 also establishes a clear medical pattern and negotiates a medical referral to a specialist. He also recognises that issues in the patient's life are complicating the situation. Near the end of the consultation, he puts it like this: *'So we've talked about quite a lot haven't we? We talked about your back pain and I'm going to refer you . . . and then we also talked about some of the stresses you've been under recently and the effects it's having on you and your relationship with your husband. And as I said before if you would like to come back another time we could talk about that some more. That's up to you.'*
This doctor recognises that there is something more complex about the issue the

RECOGNISING PATTERNS

EXPERT

- Pattern recognition is intuitive and rapid even where information is conflicting and/or inadequate.
- Confidence in own judgement.
- Ability to recognise patterns in most (complex or familiar) situations.
- Can separate patterns in complex situations and deal with each appropriately.

PROFICIENT

- Pattern recognition easier and faster but not intuitive.
- Willingness to trust own judgement.
- Shows a breadth of pattern recognition across medical, sociological and psychological domains.

COMPETENT

- Mechanistic approach.
- Varying (un)certainty in trusting own judgement.
- Recognition of serious illness patterns.
- Some appreciation of varying patient behaviour(s).

CONSULTING SKILLS

This category is about diagnostic reasoning. It relates to the processes which affect judgements and how the doctor reaches conclusions.

How to distinguish the different levels of performance

Expert
There is intuitive reasoning, a greater level of trust or distrust in the doctor's judgement. The doctor displays a greater conviction about the feelings engendered in the consultation, which in turn reinforces the reasoning process.
Proficient
Pattern recognition is faster at times, but may be mechanistic at other times. There is evidence of conscious reasoning.
Competent
The reasoning process is conscious. There is little conviction concerning the judgements made and therefore judgements are more mechanistic.

When fingerprinting, look for:

- ease and speed of hypothesis formation
- possible testing out of the hypothesis
- doctor's conviction about the hypothesis or feeling
- undisclosed evidence on fingerprint case sheet.

Recognising Patterns relates to:
- Medical Competence – where the doctor uses acquired knowledge to make decisions.
- Focus – identifying cues and clues helps the doctor to recognise patterns, and pattern recognition enables the doctor to make appropriate interventions.

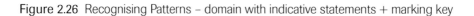

Figure 2.26 Recognising Patterns – domain with indicative statements + marking key

patient presents but thinks of it in terms of two patterns: 'backache' and 'relationship with husband'. There is a separate response to each pattern.

Doctor 3

Doctor 3 has established that the home relationship is not supportive and that the patient has no other confiding relationship. She has already explored whether she may be depressed. Towards the end of the consultation, she tests out a new hypothesis with the patient and asks her:

Doctor: *I mean, do you think how you feel and how you are is affected by the relationship – do you think it has a negative effect on your health?*

Patient: *I haven't really thought of it in those terms . . . but I suppose everything affects you at the end of the day doesn't it? Bits of your life add up to how you feel at the end of the day.*

The doctor has offered a new pattern to the patient, which she has accepted. In this pattern everything can be included with equal importance. Despite being complex, this pattern allows them to then consider the small things that can be achieved without feeling overwhelmed by the incurable chest disease and longstanding back pain, although both will need to be addressed.

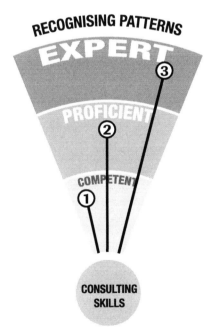

Figure 2.27 Recognising Patterns – fingerprint markings

Medical Competence – Mrs Henderson case responses

Doctor 1

Doctor 1 takes a careful history, including the medication, and establishes that the meloxicam is only partially helpful and that the patient doesn't like taking tablets. She asks whether she can have an injection. The doctor checks his understanding: *'Did you know anyone that had injections?'* and then asks after the patient has responded in the affirmative *'After injections, how long did it last for?'* The patient replies, *I think it actually resolved the situation.*

The doctor tries to persuade the patient that exercises will reduce the pain because:

Doctor: *Pain comes by spasm of the muscles, and if you don't exercise those muscles in the back they will go into even worse spasm.*

Patient: *So what you're saying is that by exercising muscles that will relieve the pain.*

Doctor: *It will relieve the pain.*

The doctor is probably correct in trying physiotherapy first, but it is not clear that he is responding to the patient's understanding. He could also have told the patient about the evidence supporting his assertion.

He offers an increase in medication and then attempts to dissuade the patient from injections:

Doctor: *If nothing helps, I wouldn't rush, if I was you, straight into injections.*

Patient: *Why?*

Doctor: *Injections – it's quite a procedure that has its own risk of infection, risk of bleeding, risk of allergy to . . . So it's not so straightforward as it seems.*

Under pressure to justify his decision to the patient, communication of risk becomes vague and unrelated to patient needs. Possibly this is because the doctor has insufficient knowledge of the true risks. Instead of admitting this and building a risk assessment into the management plan, he tries to cover up by making further assertions.

Doctor 2

As Doctor 2 outlines the possible approaches that could be taken, he does provide the patient with some evidence.

MEDICAL COMPETENCE

EXPERT

- Where appropriate, forms and challenges diagnoses, appreciates patient's understanding.
- Makes appropriate and sensitive risk assessment and responds appropriately.
- Management based firmly on up-to-date EBM principles where appropriate.
- Manages knowledge and skill gaps.
- Expertise remains functional under pressure.

PROFICIENT

- Where appropriate, can make and modify or defer diagnoses.
- Makes appropriate and sensitive risk assessment.
- Attempts to base management plan on EBM principles.
- Aware of knowledge gaps and shows some ability to address them.
- Skill sustained under pressure.

COMPETENT

- Makes appropriate diagnoses.
- Makes basic risk assessment.
- Mechanistic approach to clinical problem.
- Displays uncertainty as to knowledge and skills.
- Skills may decrease under pressure.

CONSULTING SKILLS

This area is not about judgement of medical skills; it concerns the application of acquired knowledge and skills. This includes a knowledge base of medical facts and evidence-based medicine and the necessary skills to assimilate and use them in the consultation. A key feature is the way medical skill is used and is shared with the patient.

How to distinguish the different levels of performance

Expert
> The expert has knowledge gaps, but knows where and how to address them and can show this productively in a consultation with the involvement of the patient. The expert doctor takes particular interest in the patient's viewpoint and understanding and makes quality judgements informing or challenging diagnoses. Information gathering is sensitively and efficiently achieved. Expertise may enable apparent 'flashes' or jumps to be made through skilled observation of the patient and their story.

Proficient
> A proficient doctor will gather all the necessary information and involve the patient in the consultation, but may achieve this mechanistically. The diagnoses can be made, modified or even deferred with the patient's acceptance. The doctor can cope under pressure, and has some ability to address knowledge gaps.

Competent
> A competent doctor has sufficient knowledge and skills to practice safely, albeit in a more doctor-oriented and structured fashion. The doctor's performance may display uncertainty as to their knowledge and skills and lack an evidence-based approach. If pressurised, coping mechanism may be lacking.

When fingerprinting, look for:

- involvement of the patient in the consultation
- flexibility in diagnosis and management
- self-awareness or lack of it
- how the doctor copes with pressure
- how the doctor manages knowledge/skill gaps.

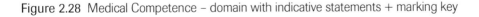

Medical Competence relates to:
- Dealing with Uncertainty – the level of uncertainty in the consultation may arise from knowledge deficiencies or even a skills shortage.
- Recognising Patterns – this category builds on the medical knowledge acquired and applies it to cases.

Figure 2.28 Medical Competence – domain with indicative statements + marking key

Doctor: . . . *some people have found them to be helpful and others don't. The negative side of the therapies is that we don't have lots and lots of studies to prove to us that they are effective. Although anecdotally, a lot of people who have tried them have found them to be effective.*

When the patient asks about injections, Doctor 2 says, '*Thinking about the injections and epidural, I'd usually go to the orthopaedic surgeons first and get them to see you and assess your back.*' The patient responds positively to the referral and then agrees to see a physiotherapist as well. Instead of placing the referrals in a sequenced management plan, the physiotherapy leading to orthopaedic referral if indicated, the doctor agrees to both.

Doctor 3

In the consultation with Doctor 3 there is the following exchange when the doctor is wondering what to do:

Doctor: *Have you ever thought about having some physio – or anything like that – on your back . . . to try and help things along?*

Patient: *Not really. It's never been put forward as an option to pursue. Not seriously anyway.*

Doctor: *And the medication you take, has it upset you in any way? Has it helped you in any way?*

Patient: *The anti-inflammatory they gave me to start with did upset my stomach but the meloxicam doesn't.*

Doctor: *And do you think they have helped to a degree?*

Patient: *They've helped to a degree but not totally, otherwise I wouldn't be here. But you know it's the fact that . . .*

Doctor: *You are struggling?*

Patient: *Yes, I am a bit.*

Notice how the doctor is feeling her way forward, taking the patient's viewpoint into consideration at each step. Important clinical information is revealed without the need for a mechanistic approach. At the end she is able to jump from the clinical to the affective realm of the patient lifeworld without losing the sense of flow in the conversation.

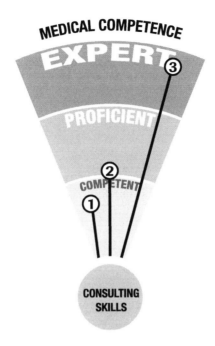

Figure 2.29 Medical Competence – fingerprint markings

Respecting Patients – Mrs Henderson case responses
Doctor 1
Doctor 1 says in relation to the backache:

Doctor: *It's restricting your life.*

Patient: *Yes.*

The doctor then moves on to ask:

Doctor: *What about socialising and time outside work? Does it interfere with your hobbies or anything else outside work?*

Patient: *Well yes, I mean even just doing things at home, you know, like cleaning the bath, I can't do any more because I can't lean to reach across. Much to my husband's disgust, I've got a cleaner.*

The doctor makes his own assumption about this and says:

Doctor: *Oh that's good.*

RESPECTING PATIENTS

EXPERT

- Shares and uses own **and** patient's ideas, concerns and expectations.
- Treats patient as equal in consultation.
- Works with the individuality of the patient.

PROFICIENT

- Accepts patient's concerns as real problems.
- Welcomes the patient on patient's terms.
- Copes with the patient and their problem(s).

COMPETENT

- Accepts patient's presenting problem(s).
- Acknowledges patient.

CONSULTING SKILLS

This area concerns the ability of the doctor to deploy their range of consulting skills to provide a strategy and choice in responding to the patient's needs.

How to distinguish the different levels of performance

Expert
There is an understanding of how the patient's problem impacts on their individual life. There is also an acknowledgement as to what the doctor and patient's perspectives are on the problem and how these can be used to help further the consultation. Valuing the patient for who they are would be the key principle in working in the expert arena.

Proficient
The proficient doctor will validate the patient's problem and attempt to get to know the patient for who they are.

Competent
The competent doctor will deal with the problem presented superficially and without any exploration of how it affects that person's life.

When fingerprinting, look for:

- how the presenting problem is dealt with: to what extent does the doctor use knowledge of what makes the patient tick in developing a management plan?
- how/if the doctor and patient share their agendas
- how the doctor manages IT aspects of the consultation.

Respecting Patients relates to:
- Communication – which is centred around establishing a common language and responding to the feelings evoked in the consultation.
- Dealing with Uncertainty – whereby the doctor's agenda is introduced and negotiated with the patient. This shared understanding provides the framework to allow working with uncertainty.

Figure 2.30 Respecting Patients – domain with indicative statements + marking key

The patient tries to correct him by saying:

Patient: *Well I think so but he's not so keen.*

The doctor doesn't pick up on this and asks a question about drugs.

He has clearly acknowledged the patient's concern as a real problem but has not worked with the individuality of the patient to explore possible solutions.

You may feel that this is an example of 'proficient' consulting. It is clearly more than minimally competent. But the proficient doctor attempts to get to know the patient for who they really are. Compare this to what Doctor 3 discovers in the example below.

Doctor 2
Doctor 2 does pick up on the comments about the husband:

Doctor: *Maybe you think you are not getting enough support from him with regards to the problem with the back.*

Patient: *Yes. Because I think that with all my other medical bits and pieces he just thinks that's one more thing . . . it's a bit of an irritant more than anything else.*

The doctor suspects an issue with the relationship and the patient confirms, '*We don't have one anymore.*' The doctor offers her the chance to talk some more but the patient declines, saying:

Patient: *I just want my back sorting out. I can sort the rest of my life out.*

The doctor accepts this but leaves a door open:

Doctor: *OK, maybe if we can get you pain-free then you can always come back to talk more if you would like to.*

This offer is repeated at the end of the consultation.

Although the doctor suspects there is something unsaid, he is willing to accept the patient perspective on the problem for the moment and keep the possibility for further exploration and discussion open.

Doctor 3
Doctor 3 starts by asking, '*Tell me why you are here.*' When the patient tells her about her backache, the first question she then asks is, '*What do you think is the root cause of it? Have you any experience of back trouble?*' The patient then says that she thinks

it started *'because I did something wrong at work.'* The doctor doesn't respond to this but later when they are discussing her chest problems she asks about her smoking. The patient replies *'. . . in all honesty I feel quite ashamed that I'm in this situation regarding (my chest).'* This time the doctor does respond to the clue and asks:

Doctor: *Why do you use the word ashamed?*

Patient: *Well it's all of my own making really isn't it, when it's boiled down to it. It's my own fault – self-inflicted.*

This has all taken place within the first two minutes of the consultation. Throughout the rest of the consultation the doctor uses her understanding of this self-blaming 'individuality' to share responsibility for addressing her problems.

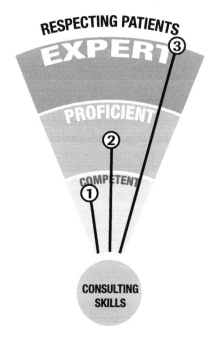

Figure 2.31 Respecting Patients – fingerprint markings

Dealing with Uncertainty – Mrs Henderson case responses
Doctor 1
Doctor 1 tells the patient at the end of the examination that *'Examining your back I think it's pretty stiff.'* He explains about muscle spasm and recommends exercise. He checks that the patient understands what he is suggesting:

DEALING WITH UNCERTAINTY

EXPERT
- In most instances obtains the patient's agreement to the use of time in making a management plan.
- Negotiates when a patient does not accept an alternative agenda.
- Explains what evidence suggests and where uncertainty and risk lie.
- Where necessary, uses uncertainty as a starting point for negotiation with patient.
- Negotiates, but sustains professional or ethical values (prepared to say 'no').

PROFICIENT
- Uses time as a diagnostic tool.
- Ensures that patient is involved in choice.
- Introduces uncertainty (with attendant risk) about diagnosis or management.
- Rarely uses interventions for which there is no evidence of effectiveness.

COMPETENT
- Attempts to involve patient in choice.
- Recognises where there is uncertainty and risk, but does not share this with patient.
- May use interventions for which there is no evidence of effectiveness.

CONSULTING SKILLS

This category considers the extent to which the doctor recognises their own and the patient's uncertainty, as well as the attendant risk, and how they act on it.

How to distinguish the different levels of performance

Expert
> The expert doctor recognises that uncertainty is the norm in medicine and integrates this into their care. In negotiations, they respect the patient's opinions, but also recognise the validity of their own views and professional and ethical values. They will use uncertainty as a diagnostic and treatment tool if applicable and deal with the remaining uncertainty in order that the patient leaves the consultation satisfied and reassured.

Proficient
> The proficient doctor not only recognises uncertainty but has come to terms with it. They will feel able to share their uncertainty with the patient. They may arrange a review to enable further information to become apparent. An evidence-based approach will almost always be used to inform treatment choices.

Competent
> The competent doctor recognises that uncertainty and risk exist, but will not appear comfortable with this. They may use the offering of choices to assure themselves, but will not share their uncertainty. This doctor will often feel a need to offer treatments even though there is insufficient evidence of the need for or effectiveness of that treatment.

When fingerprinting, look for:

- the degree to which uncertainty is mentioned in the consultation
- how/if the doctor elicits and shows understanding of the patient's beliefs and values
- how/if the doctor shares their own beliefs and values.

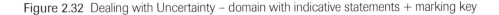

Dealing with Uncertainty relates to:
- Medical Competence – in many ways, this category is about the application of the doctor's knowledge and skills.
- Use of Resources – where there is a range of possible interventions due to the existence of uncertainty, the doctor will base their choice on the most efficient and effective ones available.

Figure 2.32 Dealing with Uncertainty – domain with indicative statements + marking key

Doctor: *Does that make sense?*

Patient: *So what you are saying is that by exercising the muscles that will relieve the pain.*

Doctor: *It will relieve the pain.*

Although the patient would like to be offered an injection which she has heard is beneficial, the doctor sticks to his plan of action. The patient's request for referral for injection is not negotiated: *'So you are thinking about injections and I am thinking about physio first. Would you be happy to think about physio and a proper range of exercise and understanding and reading something about your pain . . .'* He provides the patient with written information about exercises and arranges to review the situation in four weeks.

Notice here that while we may be influenced by the way in which this doctor is communicating with the patient, this will be addressed in another domain. Our focus here is on how he deals with uncertainty.

Doctor 2

Doctor 2 tells the patient clearly that she has sciatica and that *'consideration of orthopaedic surgeons and things like that isn't very helpful to be honest in sciatic problems unless we feel you have got a disc problem in the back.'* Now the doctor appears to become uncertain: *'But you weren't tender down the spine itself. Although you might have a bulging disc which is causing the sciatic nerve to hurt.'* The doctor does not explain how this might present a risk to the patient before offering the choice of referral to hospital. *'So one of the options would be to refer you to the hospital and they might do a scan of your back.'* The patient is referred.

Doctor 3

Doctor 3 shares her thinking with the patient throughout the consultation.

Doctor: *. . . with all your other problems as well, I think we'll have to start thinking about what we are going to have to do and to try and move things forward. There's a few things we could do.*

She explains how the early hysterectomy may have an influence on the back pain and recommends having:

Doctor: *. . . a scan of your back. We'll probably need a few blood tests doing as well I would have thought – these are routine things to see if there's . . . anything in* *the background. Then we'll have something to work on as to how we go. How does that seem?*

Patient: *Yes, I feel as if I'm making some progress.*

Later in the consultation after discussing the home situation she checks with the patient *'So is there anything else? Have we got a reasonable plan?'* She outlines the steps of the plan again and then says *'We'll get that done fairly quickly and then we can pull all that together over the next few weeks.'*

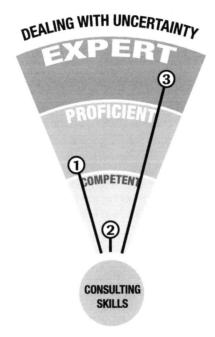

Figure 2.33 Dealing with Uncertainty – fingerprint markings

Use of Resources – Mrs Henderson case responses
Doctor 1
Doctor 1 establishes carefully the patient's expectations in relation to a diagnosis of sciatica. The patient's wish for referral conflicts with his view that physiotherapy might be appropriate. *'So you are thinking about injections and I am thinking about physio first – would you be happy to think about physio and a proper range of exercise and understanding and reading something about your pain . . .?'* He provides the patient with written information about self-care in back pain. He goes on to explain that *'injections – it's quite a procedure that has its own risks, risk of infection, risk of bleeding, risk of allergy to . . . so it's not as straightforward as it seems.'*

USE OF RESOURCES

EXPERT

• Investigation, referral, review and prescription (IRR&P) negotiated.
• Time in consultation used effectively and in negotiation with patient.
• Balances needs of individual with needs of wider community.
• Uses information sources efficiently.

PROFICIENT

• IRR&P considered and used effectively.
• Time in consultation used effectively.
• Awareness of relative cost of resources and discrimination in use.
• Uses information sources.

COMPETENT

• IRR&P done ritualistically.
• Awareness of time, but not wholly effective use of of it in consultations.
• Knows resources available, uses books, journals, protocols and IT.

CONSULTING SKILLS

This area concerns the way in which the GP doctor uses resources from health care, social care, the voluntary sector and other agencies to provide benefit to the patient. It focuses on the factors affecting the doctor's negotiating stance in relation to what is acceptable to the patient. Consideration is given to both efficiency and effectiveness of resource usage. Efficiency here is used to mean doing things economically and effectiveness means achieving the desired outcome. For example, extending a consultation and consequently avoiding unnecessary investigations is both efficient and effective.

How to distinguish the different levels of performance

Expert
> The expert doctor will achieve an agreed management plan using only those resources that clearly benefit the patient (even if it means compromising efficiency and/or effectiveness) and will have given consideration to the issue of limited health resources.

Proficient
> The proficient doctor demonstrates consideration of the relative value of all resources used to help the patient, particularly in use of time in the consultation.

Competent
> The competent doctor will use resources predominantly according to rules, whether such application is appropriate or not.

When fingerprinting, look for:

• negotiation of interventions on the basis of patient acceptability
• clear statements of value and risk (usually evidence-based) to aid patient understanding.

NB. This domain may be difficult to mark because of the different areas covered by indicative statements – evaluative tensions may arise between the different areas. Too detailed a concentration on individual resource elements may cause confusion. It is therefore acceptable to make an overall judgement based on professional experience.

Use of Resources relates to:
• Dealing with Uncertainty – where uncertainty exists the doctor will use information about the resources available to devise the most appropriate management plan.
• Synthesising Skills – whereby the doctor balances their needs and the patient's to achieve a consensual management plan.
• Focus - both categories identify the importance of making interventions in terms of the wider community and achieving concordance.

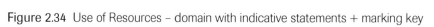

Figure 2.34 Use of Resources – domain with indicative statements + marking key

While we may disagree with the way this doctor presents his argument – that lies within the Respect for Patients domain – it is clear that he is attempting to make best use of resources and implies an understanding of the evidence base.

Doctor 2

Doctor 2 offers a number of treatment options to the patient, the last being referral for an orthopaedic assessment. '*And then there's consideration of orthopaedic surgeons and things like that, which isn't terribly helpful to be honest in sciatic problems unless we feel you've got a disc problem in the back. But you weren't tender down the spine itself.*' The doctor is beginning to think aloud and continues: '*Although you might have a bulging disc there which is causing the sciatic nerve to hurt. So one of the options would be to refer you to the hospital and they might do a scan on your back.*' The doctor offers the patient the choice and the patient gratefully accepts referral.

In addition, this doctor offers alternative therapies and alters medication. While each action may be appropriate, we can wonder whether everything has to be offered and implemented at once in an unstructured way.

Doctor 3

The consultation with Doctor 3 takes a longer time, over 20 minutes. During this time she and the patient discuss the back problem and how it is affecting home life and work. They make plans for managing the COPD and discuss how the hysterectomy 'early in life' may be contributing to the back pain. The doctor explains that there are a number of tests that could be done, including basic blood tests, hormone tests and bone scans for bone density and possible disc problems. She sums it all up like this:

Doctor: *We'll probably need a few blood tests doing as well I would have thought to see if there's anything in the background. Then we'll have something to work on as to how we go . . . it may get to the point eventually (where) you have to see a specialist but unless we've sorted a few things out and tried a few things there's no way surgeons or what have you like to start interfering . . . I think we need to be fairly clear about what the problem is.*

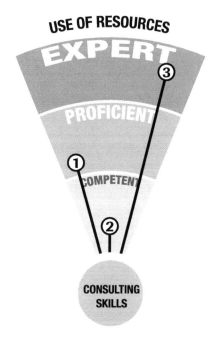

Figure 2.35 Use of resources – fingerprint markings

Focus – Mrs Henderson case responses
Doctor 1
Doctor 1 takes a traditional medical approach to the consultation. He starts by asking what is 'the problem'. The first 10 minutes of the consultation are all about the physical back pain. It appears to be a focused consultation. At 11 minutes he asks the patient:

Doctor:	*How do you otherwise feel in yourself?*
Patient:	*Not too bad.*
Doctor:	*Not too bad?*
Patient:	*Well with everything else.*
Doctor:	*Everything else?*
Patient:	*With the problems, you know, you were asking about. What I can do and all the rest of it – obviously my back is causing a problem but that with my chest as well . . . two things together are not ideal by any means.*

The doctor has been using communication skills effectively but does not respond to the cue about chest problems. Instead he asks, '*Do you have any other stresses in your life?*' The doctor is interested in exploring the patient's psychological well-being, but the consultation is focused on the presented clinical problem in such a way that it is impossible to shift the focus away from the doctor's agenda. The opportunity to include the chest problems in the discussion is passed.

FOCUS

EXPERT

- All interventions appropriate to immediate and wider context.
- Involves patient in understanding management options in all problem areas.
- Sustains clarity whilst dealing with multiple problems.
  - Uses cues and clues sensitively.
    - Able to shift focus productively.

PROFICIENT

- Majority of interventions appropriate to immediate and wider context.
  - Prioritises problems and deals with them in order of importance.
- Multi-tasking – handles some but not all problems.
- Responds to cues, and some clues, appropriately.

COMPETENT

- Some interventions appropriate to presenting problem.
  - May have a disorganised approach to multi-tasking.
    - Reacts to events.
    - Clues and cues may not always be identified or addressed.

CONSULTING SKILLS

*cues = information, verbal or non-verbal, that must be addressed.
**clues = potentially relevant information.

This category is about keeping the patient's and the doctor's agendas in mind and ensuring they are addressed to the full. The doctor's agenda includes computer-generated clinical and organisational prompts.

How to distinguish the different levels of performance

Expert
The doctor notes cues and clues,** but addresses them at the most appropriate stage of the consultation in order to ensure that as many ideas as possible are expressed and explored.

Proficient
The doctor is able to see beyond the expressed needs of the patient and deals with problems as they are presented by the patient or as they occur to the consulter.

Competent
The doctor meets the expressed needs of the patient, but may do so in a disorganised fashion.

When fingerprinting, look for:

- the depth to which the presenting problem(s) are explored
- the extent to which the doctor introduces their agenda
- how the cues are followed up
- how multiple problems are dealt with.

Focus relates to:

- Synthesising Skills/Responding Flexibly – after establishing the focus of the consultation, the doctor then selects which approach to employ.
- Communication – here the doctor will select from the cues* that they have identified and use them sensitively.
- Medical Competence – because a lack of knowledge will lead to agenda items being overlooked or insufficiently addressed.

Figure 2.36 Focus – domain with indicative statements + marking key

Doctor 2

Like Doctor 1, Doctor 2 identifies fewer problems in the consultation compared to Doctor 3. This makes it easier to keep the problem of 'back pain' as the central issue of the consultation. While the doctor discusses the home relationship quite fully, this is in the context of 'the backache': *'And how are things going? Having a lot of pain can create stress at home.'* When it is clear that there are issues at home, the doctor offers the patient support for this but moves back to the backache when support is declined. However, at the end of the consultation the doctor repeats that the offer of support is still available.

Doctor 2 misses a cue in the following sequence when the patient says:

Patient: *I just want to move, to be able to move about a bit more. The other problems I've got stop me moving a lot anyway.*

Doctor: *What problems are those?*

Patient: *Just the breathing issue.*

Doctor: *The COPD, yeh?*

Patient: *So I'm in a difficult position really. Can't move a lot anyway.*

The doctor interprets this as referring to the back and says:

Doctor: *So I'm going to need to examine you – examine your back.*

The chest problem is not discussed further in the consultation. Nor is the cue that the husband doesn't share the car (not mentioned previously). So the doctor appears to hold focus by not exploring whether another priority needs to be considered.

Doctor 3

Doctor 3 establishes a whole range of issues relating to the patient's health. She signals what she is doing:

Doctor: *Now obviously the other main problem you have looking back is the chest that you've got. That's obviously been giving you a lot of trouble over the last few months . . .*

Then she checks that she understands whether she needs to consider this as a priority:

Doctor: *Now you've seen the specialist regarding that haven't you? How's the treatment going with that because you've had one or two adjustments . . .?*

This doctor establishes from the notes that the patient has had a hysterectomy and has an HRT implant. She does not discuss this further until she discusses management options with the patient. When she does discuss management options, she outlines options in each of the problem areas: shortness of breath, pain and immobility from the back, and an unsupportive home relationship.

Notice how, in the example given in Medical Competence, when the patient describes her lifeworld, the doctor is able to 'go there'. This doctor places the focus on the complex lifeworld situation of the patient, not just on the clinical problems.

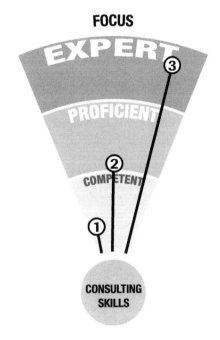

Figure 2.37 Focus – fingerprint markings

Synthesising Skills – Mrs Henderson case response
Doctor 1
Doctor 1 takes a doctor-centred approach to the back pain. His recommendation of exercises and self-help is evidence-based, but he does not explain this to the patient nor does he negotiate alternative approaches. When the patient clearly wishes to do something different (have a spinal injection), he has no alternative approach that could include her preferences in the management plan.

Doctor 2
Doctor 2 quickly realises that there are important issues in the patient's home life

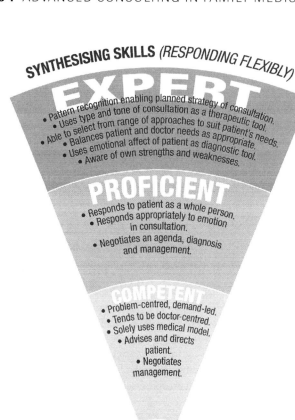

This area concerns the ability of the doctor to deploy their range of consulting skills to provide a holistic strategy and choice in responding to the patient's needs.

How to distinguish the different levels of performance

Expert
The expert doctor can adapt from a range of approaches to suit the patient's needs: what sort of doctor should s/he be, what sort of patient should the patient be? The interaction of the relationship may be used for diagnostic as well as therapeutic means. A high degree of self-knowledge may be required to interpret and make beneficial use of the messages arising from the relationship.

Proficient
The doctor can see the presenting problem within the context of the whole patient, their life, environment and ongoing problems. The doctor may respond to other messages arising from the patient's behaviour, recognising that the patient's needs may be more complex than the immediate solution to the presenting problem. In this case, the agenda for both the consultation and the management will be negotiated.

Competent
The doctor is able to identify the presenting problem, make a diagnosis and negotiate a management plan.

When fingerprinting, look for:

- evidence of choices being made from a range of possible responses
- a recognition of the reasons for the choices negotiated and made.

 Synthesising Skills/Responding Flexibly relates to:
- Synthesising Skills/Responding Flexibly is the application of all the other categories..

Figure 2.38 Synthesising Skills with indicative statements + marking key

that may be relevant to the backache but approaches them as issues separate from the backache. The doctor responds to clues and enquires about each issue in turn. The patient, however, may not have understood how all the issues relate: *'If I wasn't so uncomfortable I would feel better – you know – coping with everything. Even the little things, like I said about getting to work, I go on the bus because he has the car. I could do with having the car . . . if I wasn't poorly it wouldn't be an issue.'*

The doctor is therefore unable to negotiate a management plan that covers all aspects of the patient's needs at the same time.

Doctor 3

Doctor 3 establishes that there are many elements to the patient's backache and treats them all together as a complex issue. She has already included more issues than the other doctors: smoking and COPD, previous hysterectomy, relationship with husband and work, as well as establishing the way the patient feels about herself (*'It's my own fault – self inflicted'*). The doctor outlines possible ways forward for each issue but also puts the whole complex issue before the patient: *'I mean do you think – how you feel and how you are, is affected by the relationship – do you think it has a negative effect on your health?'*

As a result of doing this, she is later able to shift strategy and engage the patient in the implementation of their agreed plan:

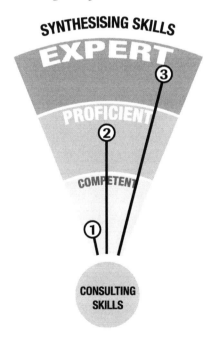

Figure 2.39 Synthesising Skills – fingerprint markings

Doctor: *I guess you have to start somewhere, try to change things. There's you involved in it and obviously there are some things outside your control but I guess there are things that you can try to do for yourself and we'll try and play our part. And there's your social setting and your husband and work and they all fit together in some way. Don't they? So is there anything else? Have we got a reasonable plan?*

Patient: *Yes, I feel as though I am taking a step forward.*

ADVANCED CONSULTING – A SUMMARY

The Consultation Expertise Model provides a means for detailed identification of expertise progression to an advanced level. In endeavouring to sum up ways in which expert doctors consult, we advocate that expertise at this high level can be encapsulated by the following four attributes:

ATTRIBUTES OF ADVANCED CONSULTING

Advanced consulting can be identified by outcomes that are:

❏ **Fluent** – as with all expert behaviour, it looks easy and appears to be seamless, and because of this, it is difficult to detect its constituent parts. Fluency implies speed of perception and decision making and as such means that more information can be obtained in the same time span. New doctors may feel little is happening while watching an expert at work. In fact, complex *nondescript processes* are occurring.

'The most experienced physicians' cognitive task diagrams reflected not detailed descriptions but extremely general, almost nondescript processes which in their generality encompassed great flexibility.'[65]

'One of the most fascinating aspects of people with high levels of personal mastery is their ability to accomplish extraordinary complex tasks with grace and ease.'[66]

❏ **Holistic** – interaction with the patient is contextualised in medical, social, emotional and psychological terms for that moment in time and for the future. In this sense expert consultations may be considered to be more *complete*. The observable outcome of a holistic approach is *completeness*.

ATTRIBUTES OF ADVANCED CONSULTING

'The traditional expectation is that expert decisions are made by explicit evaluation of alternatives on the basis of comparison of salient elements. But in actuality, expert decisions are more holistic.'[67]

❏ **Flexible** – because the expert is, by definition, more experienced and therefore has a wider repertoire of interpersonal skill and perception, they can manage a wide range of case challenges successfully whilst managing their own personal anxieties. Flexibility implies that a doctor can *start anywhere* in the consultation in response to the patient and still achieve *completeness*.

'Personal mastery goes beyond competence and skills, though it is grounded in competence and skills . . . It means approaching one's life as a creative work, living life from a creative as opposed to reactive viewpoint.'[68]

❏ **Proactive** – because the expert has *been there before* it is more possible to anticipate and find creative ways of handling difficult situations. This is helped by heuristics (rules of thumb)[69] and maxims.

'The art of selecting the most appropriate medical maxim for a particular decision is acquired largely through the accumulation of "case expertise" (the stories or "illness scripts" of patients and clinical anecdotes).'[70]

References

1. Spence J. *The Purpose and Practice of Medicine*. Oxford: Oxford University Press; 1960.
2. WONCA Europe. *The European Definition of General Practice/Family Medicine*; 2002. Available at: www.euract.org/page03f.html (accessed 8 August 2008).
3. RCGP. *Curriculum for Speciality Training for General Practice, The Core Statement: being a general practitioner*. London: Royal College of General Practitioners; 2007.
4. Harrison J, Innes R, van Zwanenberg T. *The New GP*. Oxford: Radcliffe Medical Press; 2000. p. 32.
5. Mamede S, Schmidt H, Rickers R, *et al.* Breaking down automaticity: case ambiguity

and the shift to reflective approaches in clinical reasoning. *Med Educ.* 2002; **41**(12): 1185–92.

6. Eraut M. *Developing Professional Knowledge and Competence.* London: Falmer Press; 1994.

7. Heyrman J. *Consequences of Learning Concepts to Programs and Curricula in General Practice* [as Personal Communication], 2005.

8. Benner P. *From Novice to Expert: excellence and power in clinical nursing practice.* New Jersey: Prentice Hall; 1984.

9. Eraut, op cit. p. 123.

10. Coderre S, Mandin H, Harasym P, *et al.* Diagnostic reasoning strategies and diagnostic success. *Med Educ.* 2003; **37**: 695–703.

11. Elwyn G. *Shared Decision Making: patient involvement in clinical practice.* Nijmegan: WOK; 2001. p. 15.

12. Sweeney K. *Complexity in Primary Care.* Oxford: Radcliffe Medical Press; 2006. p. 37.

13. Eraut, op cit. p.125.

14. Medawar PB. *Induction and Intuition in Scientific Thought.* London: Methuen; 1969. p. 43.

15. Zeldin T. *Conversation: how talk can change our lives.* London: Hidden Spring; 1998. p. 1.

16. Polanyi M. *The Tacit Dimension.* London: Routledge; 1967.

17. Hargie O, editor. *The Handbook of Communication Skills.* 3rd ed. London: Routledge; 2006. p. 8.

18. Innes AD, Campion PD, Griffiths FE. Complex consultations and the 'edge of chaos'. *Br J Gen Pract.* 2005; **55**(510): 47–52.

19. Salinsky J, Sackin P. *What Are You Feeling Doctor?* Oxford: Radcliffe Medical Press; 2000. p. 11.

20. Eraut M. *Factors Affecting Workplace Learning in the Workplace: providing grassroots for learning organisations.* Handout for presentation to the Centre for Labour Market Studies. University of Leicester; 2006

21. Norfolk T. *Developing the Personal Competencies of GP Registrars: new training modules.* London: City University; 2004. p. 5.

22. Greenhalgh T, Hurwitz B. *Narrative Based Medicine.* London: BMJ Books; 1998. p. xiii.

23. Kurtz S, Silverman J, Draper J. *Teaching and Learning Communication Skills in Medicine.* Oxford: Radcliffe Medical Press; 1998. p. 13.

24. Janacek L (1928) quoted in an Opera North programme for Janacek's opera *Katya Kabanova*; 2007. p. 18.

25. Elstein G, Schwarts A. Clinical problem-solving and diagnostic decision making. *BMJ.* 2002; **324**: 729–32.

26. Gladwell M. *Blink: the power of thinking without thinking.* London: Penguin-Allen Lane; 2005. p. 23.

27. Schmidt H, Norman G, Boshuizen A. A cognitive perspective on medical expertise: theory and expectations. *Acad Med.* 1990; **65**: 10.

28. Sackett D, *et al.* Evidence based medicine: What it is and what it isn't. *BMJ* 1996; **312**: 71–2.

29. Sweeney, op cit. p. 43.

30. Ashton L, Worrall P. Going there. *Educ Prim Care.* 2008; **19**: 84–9.

31. Gillet G. Medical science, culture, and truth. *Philos Ethics Humanit Med.* 2006; **1**: 1–13.

32. GMC. *Good Medical Practice.* London: General Medical Council; 2006.

33. Barry C, Stevenson F, Britten N, *et al.* Giving voice to the lifeworld. More humane, more effective medical care? A qualitative study of doctor-patient communication in general practice. *Soc Sci Med.* 2001; **53**: 487–505.

34. Barry, *et al.,* op cit.

35. Rogers C. *On Becoming a Person: a therapist's view of psychotherapy.* London: Constable; 1967. p. 282.

36. Elwyn G, Edwards A, Kinnersley P. Shared decision-making in primary care: the neglected second half of the consultation. *Br J Gen Pract.* 1999; **49**: 477–82.

37. Levinson W. Physician-patient communication: a key to malpractice prevention. *JAMA.* 1994; **272**: 1619–20.

38. Goodman K. *Ethics and Evidence Based Medicine.* Cambridge: Cambridge University Press; 2003. p. 139.

39. Leader D, Corfield D. *Why Do Patients Get Ill?* London: Hamish Hamilton; 2007.

40. Scarborough H. *The Management of Expertise.* Basingstoke: Macmillan Business; 1996.

41. Helman C. *Suburban Shaman: tales from medicine's front line.* London: Hammersmith Press; 2006.

42. Mead N, Bower P. Patient-centredness: a conceptual framework and review of empirical literature. *Soc Sci Med.* 2000; **51**: 1087–110.

43. McDonald CJ. Medical heuristics: the silent adjudicators of clinical practice. *Ann Inter Med.* 1996; **124**(1 Pt.1): 56–62.

44. Schön D. *Educating the Reflective Practitioner.* San Francisco: Jossey-Bass; 1987. p. 5.

45. Endsley M, Garland D. *Situation Awareness Analysis and Measurement.* Mahwah, NJ: Lawrence Erlbaum Associates Inc.; 2000.

46. Endsley M. Towards a theory of situational awareness in dynamic systems. *Hum Factors.* 1995; **37**(1): 32–64.

47. Senge P, Scharmer CO, Jaworski J, *et al. Presence: exploring profound change*

in people, organisations and society. London: Nicholas Brealey Publishing; 2005. pp. 13–15.

48. Eraut, op cit. p. 112.
49. Bloom B, Krathwohl DR, *et al. Taxonomy of Educational Objectives: Handbook 1 Cognitive Domain.* London: Longman Group; 1956. p. 206.
50. Medawar PB. *Induction and Intuition in Scientific Thought.* London: Methuen; 1969. p. 46.
51. Sackett D, Richardson SR, Rosenberg W, *et al. Evidence Based Medicine.* 2nd ed. Edinburgh: Churchill-Livingstone 1997. p. 1.
52. Medawar, op cit. p. 46.
53. Medawar, op cit. p. 59.
54. A personal communication from Good D quoted by Wakeford R. In: Commentary: criteria, competences, and confidence tricks. *BMJ.* 2006; **332**(28): 233.
55. Eraut, op cit. p. 145.
56. www.rcgp.org.uk/docs/nMRCGP_COT_Guide_to_Performance_Criteria.doc (accessed 24 October 2008).
57. Dreyfus H, Dreyfus S. *Mind over Machine: the power of human intuition and expertise in the era of the computer.* New York: Free Press; 1986.
58. Michael Eraut. *Developing Professional Knowledge and Competence.* London: Falmer Press; 1994. p. 124.
59. www.rcgp-curriculum.org.uk/examinations_and_assessment.aspx (accessed 28 October 2008)
60. Dreyfus, Dreyfus, op cit. p. 36.
61. Ibid. p. 28.
62. Ibid. p. 30.
63. www.rcgp-curriculum.org.uk/rcgp_-_gp_curriculum_documents/gp_curriculum_statements.aspx (accessed 24 October 2008).
64. www.rcgp-curriculum.org.uk/nmrgcp/wpba/consultation_observation_tool.aspx (accessed 28 October 2008).
65. Christenson R. Fetters M, Green L. Opening the black box: cognitive strategies in family practice. *Ann Fam Med.* 2005; **3**(2).
66. Senge P. *The Fifth Discipline: the art and practice of the learning organisation.* New York: Doubleday; 1990.
67. Benner, op cit.
68. Senge, Scharmer, Jaworski, op cit.
69. McDonald C. Medical heuristics: the silent adjudicators of practice. *Ann Intern Med.* 1996; **124**(1 Pt. 1): 56–62.
70. Greenhalgh T. Narrative based medicine in an evidence based world. *BMJ.* 1999; **318**: 323–5.

3 FINGERPRINTING

Fingerprints using the Consultation Expertise Model provide an interpretation of single or multiple family doctor cases.

- Impression Graph
- Making a fingerprint
- Common marking problems
- Giving fingerprint feedback

FINGERPRINT PACK

Downloadable paperwork (*see* Appendix 4)

The pack contains:

- ❑ Patient Consent Form
- ❑ Conditions Governing Tapes
- ❑ Fingerprint Case Sheet
- ❑ Impression Graph Sheet
- ❑ Domains – Indicative Statements
- ❑ Six Case Fingerprint Sheet (Pro Forma)
- ❑ Six Case Impression Graph
- ❑ Feedback Guidance
- ❑ Feedback Sheets 1 And 2
- ❑ Reflection Sheet

THE IMPRESSION GRAPH

The Consultation Expertise Model uses two visual components in the recording of consultations: the eight-domain *fingerprint* and the four-bar *Impression Graph*.

The Impression Graph – how it emerged

The purpose of the Model is to help us with our understanding and development of

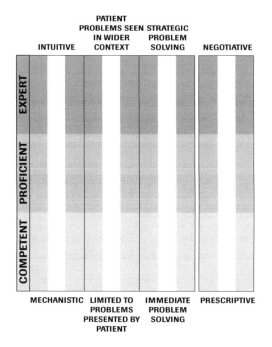

Figure 3.01 The Impression Graph

expertise. We need therefore to understand how we differentiate between expertise and non-expertise.

The Impression Graph emerged in response to the question: how can we classify our understanding of the characteristics of the competent, proficient and expert doctor?

In academic terms, is it possible to provide a typology of the three performance levels to assist users' understanding of the Model? Without such an understanding of the difference between the three performance levels, the Model is incomplete.

> 'If some aspects of professional practice cannot be readily defined, quantified or observed, they cannot easily be assessed [formatively in our case] by conventional means. The result is likely to be that they are not valued.'[1]

The fingerprint encapsulates the specific behaviours that can be observed at each of the three performance levels in each domain, but it does not provide an analysis or overview of the attributes of each performance level.

The Impression Graph allows analysis of the consultation according to four broad themes:
- acting intuitively
- engaging with patients' lifeworld

- thinking strategically
- negotiation.

Each of the four themes is presented as a differential on a sliding scale. The first three themes are linked sequentially. Strategic thinking will be dependent upon understandings gained from engagement with the patient's lifeworld. The need for such engagement is in turn dependent upon intuition. The fourth bar, *negotiative/ prescriptive*, is deliberately separate from the others, as there will be consultations where the process is of necessity more prescriptive than negotiated (such as a high level of suspicion of a cancer or where a patient makes it clear they want the doctor to take control of decisions), whereas flexibility within the other bars occurs more readily in any consultation.

Thinking in terms of the four themes allows a rapid judgement to be made of the consultation as a whole. The linkage of the themes allows a preliminary check of this judgement. It is unlikely that expertise will be demonstrated in terms of strategic thinking unless a similar level of expertise has been demonstrated in the other two themes.

The Impression Graph has two purposes

Not only does the Impression Graph provide a conceptual overview, it also has a marking role. It is customary in marking where a judgement or value threshold plays a significant part to juxtapose detailed marking, represented by the indicative statements, with more subjective, holistic impression marking in order to correlate a final judgement. The Impression Graph therefore serves as an adjunct to the indicative statements in the fingerprinting process.

The place of the Impression Graph in the Consultation Expertise Model

The dimensions of the Impression Graph are consistent with the Dreyfus typology we had started with (*see* p. 61).

The progression from mechanistic/standardised to intuitive/tacit is also consistent with the nature of expertise development. It is because these underpinning interpersonal, problem-solving and medical skills become second nature that expert consulting may look deceptively easy. Higher-order thinking by experts cannot be as readily observed when compared with doctors who work explicitly to rules and guidelines.

> '*The two highest levels of skill . . . are characterised by a rapid, fluid, involved kind of behaviour that bears no similarity to the slow, detached reasoning of the problem-solving process.*'[2]

The dimensions concerned with seeing patient problems in their wider strategic context do not mirror Dreyfus statements because they are specific to family medicine; however they do link with the language of holism and concordance and the need to take an overview (*see* Concordance, p.158). In a similar way, the *Negotiative/Prescriptive* dimension contains a specifically medical understanding.

Using the Impression Graph for fingerprinting

It is customary to complete the Impression Graph before going on to fingerprinting domains. As mentioned in the following chapter, completing the diagram is comparatively easy and reflects an 'overall feeling' about the consultation. However, finding words to support that 'feeling' can be difficult. Experience has shown that completing the written section of the Impression Graph is often made easier after considering the detailed behaviours identified for the fingerprint.

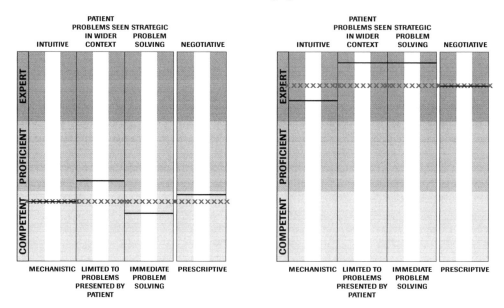

Figure 3.02 Impression Graph capture of expertise for two doctors consulting with the same patient simulation

The Impression Graph can be seen to provide an 'at a glance' level of expertise.

Approaches to Impression Graph marking

The following ideas may be of help when completing an Impression Graph:
1.   Column one
     —   How does the consultation start (experts can **start anywhere**) and how easy does it look? Fluency is a marker of intuitive behaviour. It should be

easy to observe whether the consultation starts with the doctor's agenda or with one of the many threads that are more to do with establishing rapport and the patient's agenda.

2. Column two
   — Does the consultation **go there**? It is usually clear when the consultation moves into the lifeworld of the patient. Consultations lacking lifeworld information are sometimes incomplete so limiting the strategic thinking required for column 3.

3. Column three
   — Is the doctor thinking and acting **proactively**, as evidenced by empathetic explanation, the use of communication aids that indicate the doctor has previous experience of patients' difficulty with a condition? Proactive action is a likely response to pattern recognition. Equally important is the doctor thinking ahead on behalf of the patient using the information gained from a full history, i.e. thinking strategically.

4. Column four
   — Is the consultation **concordant**? This is a helpful concept for spotting genuine negotiation and shared understanding.

It is important to complete the Impression Graph immediately after watching the consultation in order to capture an 'impression' of the performance level. This can then be compared with the more detailed marking of the fingerprint. Juxtaposing a subjective impression mark with a detailed marking schema is a customary marking procedure designed to produce well-considered judgements in higher education.

Interesting graphs arise when one area in the first of the three dimensions stands out because it is out of line with the others; for example, some people have difficulty with the notion of intuition and are therefore wary of marking this dimension highly. In a single consultation there may be a good reason for this, but if this recurred over several consultations it will indicate a matter for the marker, not the consulter.

A line of 'best fit' drawn across the Impression Graph as an overall judgement of the case performance level, as in Figure 3.02 above, will provide a performance locator to compare with the fingerprint pattern. If there is a serious or non-explainable discrepancy, the marking needs to be reconsidered.

The Impression Graph provides one means of identifying and valuing consultations at all performance levels.

MAKING A FINGERPRINT
The purpose of fingerprinting
Fingerprinting is a form of marking. It is a technique integrally associated with the

Consultation Expertise Model and made technically possible early in the project development because the domains were designed on a circular basis. The fingerprint is used to mark consultations for personal reflection, feedback for self-interested development or appraisal and revalidation purposes. **The purpose of fingerprinting is to assist development of family doctor consulting skill, stage by stage, in known contexts.** The project group is adamant that fingerprinting should not be considered or used for any kind of summative assessment. It is anticipated that fingerprinting contexts will range from that of a family doctor registrar in the final months of training, to a family doctor trainer fingerprinting his or her consultations for educational purposes or to serving doctors making fingerprints for personal reflection, for appraisal or maybe for use as evidence for revalidation.

The new doctor who enters practice at the level of competence or above can integrate fingerprinting into his or her practice from the start on the assumption that higher levels of skill will occur as experience grows, **if that experience is 'deliberative'**, that is, incorporating a self-conscious, intentional desire to benefit from experience using reflection. A key principle of reflective practice is the use of external reference points from literature, journals, patient and colleague feedback etc.

The context will be different for a family doctor who has not previously recorded consultations. There may be sensitivity exposing what is normally only shared with patients to colleague eyes, maybe leaving the 'comfort zone', or practical issues regarding recording equipment and consent forms.

The fingerprint provides a means to identify performance stages on the competent to expert continuum in eight domains **on a case-by-case basis**. Experience of using the model has shown that some family doctor registrars will, towards the end of training, be capable of performing at *proficient* levels in some domains – they respond to the needs of the case. It is important to acknowledge this because confidence is a major factor in gaining benefit from experience. Being able to identify and affirm this in specific terms can not only be rewarding but also reinforce the notion of progression. Conversely, because fingerprints are case-specific, a well-experienced doctor may register *competent* simply because the case was undemanding or because other variables were affecting the consultation.

Reminder – assumptions underpinning the Model

When fingerprinting, it is important to bear in mind some of the assumptions made by the group when they developed the Model.

- It is assumed throughout that higher-order consulting is associated with better health outcomes.
- The Model is a formative tool. It has not been designed, nor is it valid, for assessment.

- The Model is designed to look at higher levels of expertise, not basic skills.
- The Model should not be used for family doctors in training until they are sufficiently competent.
- Expert doctors cannot be expected to perform consistently at a higher level because:
  — the case may not provide sufficient opportunity, i.e. challenge, to employ higher-level skills.
  — personal and/or external variables may affect the doctor/patient interaction.

Practicalities – making a fingerprint

For the consulter

Stage 1 – Preparation

- Decide how the fingerprint will be used. Will it be for private reflection or dialogue with colleagues?
- How will it be recorded – by camera or by observation?
- If the consultation is to be seen by others, or there is to be an exchange of tapes, make sure the *Conditions Governing Tapes* sheet is signed (*see* p. 207).
- Either arrange for the observer or set up the recording equipment. Think ahead – will your type of recording equipment be compatible with that of colleagues' for playback?
- Arrange with reception staff to gain patients' consent to recording and complete the first part of the consent form (in the Fingerprint Pack). Some practices have already adopted online booking, which bypasses reception, leaving the doctor to complete both parts of the Consent Form.
- Record consultation(s).
- Fill in the *Fingerprint Case Sheet* (*see* p. 208), noting particularly those things that were in your mind that will not be observable on the recording. This will be particularly important with patients you are familiar with. Decide on the status of case challenge, a major variable when interpreting the fingerprint.

CASE CHALLENGE

A = Straightforward clinical case.
B = More complex clinical case.
C = A clinical or psychological or combined clinical psychological case that *challenges* the doctor.

For the fingerprinter

Stage 2a – Fingerprinting a recorded consultation

Before reading this section scan the paperwork provided in the Fingerprint Pack – Appendix 4.

- Read the Fingerprint Case Sheet.
- View the consultation, making a mental or written note of significant moments. Significant moments are those times when a consultation changes direction, e.g. when response to a cue prompts the patient to disclose important issues. Alternatively, when you are familiar with the Model, use the Feedback Sheet to act as an aide-memoir for feedback.
- Rate the consultation on the four differentials of the Impression Graph, and draw a line across the graph as a mean of the four marks in order to establish a generalised performance level.
- Use the indicative statements in all eight domains to produce a case fingerprint.
    - Use **NA** (not applicable) if it is not appropriate to mark a domain.
    - There are seven dots in each domain. Mark to the dots. Dot 1 indicates less than competent. Dots 3-5-7 indicate the three performance levels, and dots 2-4-6 the 'not sure' points within each performance level. *Think of the pond-dipping analogy (see Figure 2.23, p. 69) and the balance of frogspawn, tadpoles and frogs to assist with the surety of decisions.* (Those familiar with marking may use more freehand marks by ignoring the dots.)
    - Be guided by the indicative statements – 'did you see this happen?'
    - As you decide the mark for each domain, record observations and comments on the Feedback Sheet.
    - When all eight domains are marked, review the case challenge A-B-C judgement and record your decision on the Fingerprint Case Sheet.
    - Review the finished fingerprint – 'what does it show?' Compare the fingerprint with the Impression Graph generalised performance line. If there is a discrepancy, rethink the marking and adjust the marks so that there is agreement between both sheets.

There are helpful marking notes for each domain. To reinforce these, the following single points might aid interpretation:

- Communication – interpersonal skills and person-to-person understandings in use – is the quality of rapport maintained throughout the consultation?
- Recognising Patterns – is there evidence of pattern recognition regarding patient characteristics as well as clinical condition?

- Medical Competence – remember that it is the application of medical knowledge and skill that characterises this domain.
- Dealing with Uncertainty – is uncertainty made explicit and discussed or utilised with the patient?
- Respecting Patients – at what level is there engagement with and consideration for the individuality of the patient?
- Use of Resources – an overall impression of usage of time; evaluation of cost; effectiveness of resources employed; and involvement of the patient as a resource.
- Focus – to what extent was a complete patient picture obtained and dealt with?
- Synthesising Skills – did the Fingerprint Case Sheet indicate a strategy seen on the recording? Was the consultation summarised and shared with the patient?
- Decide on issues for feedback, remembering specifically to include areas requested by the consulter for feedback.

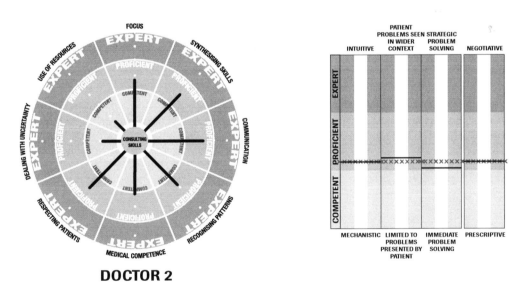

DOCTOR 2

Figure 3.03 Marked Impression Graph alongside a fingerprint of the same case

Stage 2b – Fingerprinting an observed consultation

Decide the priority areas beforehand. Do you want to consider all the domains or concentrate on specific domains? Are you interested in developing specific behaviours reflected in specific indicative statements? Do you have a particular focus, e.g. 'What expertise can I employ if I stick to a 10-minute consultation?'

Record significant or relevant observations as the consultation progresses. Match these with the indicative statements post-consultation.

or

Use the Impression Graph dimensions as a working discussion framework.

Stage 2c – Multiple-case fingerprinting (Figure 3.04)

A fingerprint of a single case will provide detailed evidence for a feedback dialogue, a dialogue that will have extra resonance if the consultation has been chosen by the doctor with specific feedback needs in mind. More informative, albeit requiring more effort to fingerprint, may be a choice of six consultations from a normal surgery list. If the chosen six include a range of A-C case challenges and kind (e.g. chronic, acute, young, old), the resultant series of fingerprints can give a good overall picture of the doctor's consulting behaviour. This can be particularly interesting with experienced doctors when fingerprints range from competent to expert in relation to case challenge and which indicate expert behaviour in different domains from case to case. No one in our experience has recorded expert behaviour in all eight domains on one consultation. This seems to be totally unrealistic. Nevertheless, a doctor might achieve expert level in all domains over a sequence of cases, thus showing overall expert capability. Alternatively, a doctor may show expertise in some domains and not in others, thus presenting a significant feedback opportunity.

Stage 3 – Feedback discussion

- Confirm what specific feedback the colleague wants in relation to expertise in general or priority areas.
- Provide feedback according to Consultation Expertise Model Feedback Guidance. (*Fingerprint Pack* in Appendix 4).
- Hold dialogue – consider what has been learned.
- Complete Reflection Sheet.
- Record learning and future practice needs on a learning plan.
- Make an action plan – how will these needs be addressed?

COMMON MARKING PROBLEMS

General points to be born in mind when using the Model to fingerprint are:

- It should not be assumed that collections of indicative statements in any domain in themselves represent the total sum of any performance level – performance cannot be reduced in this way. The Model is designed for dialogue and development of expertise, not for definitive marking.
- Indicative statements are just that – indicative. Expect each doctor to

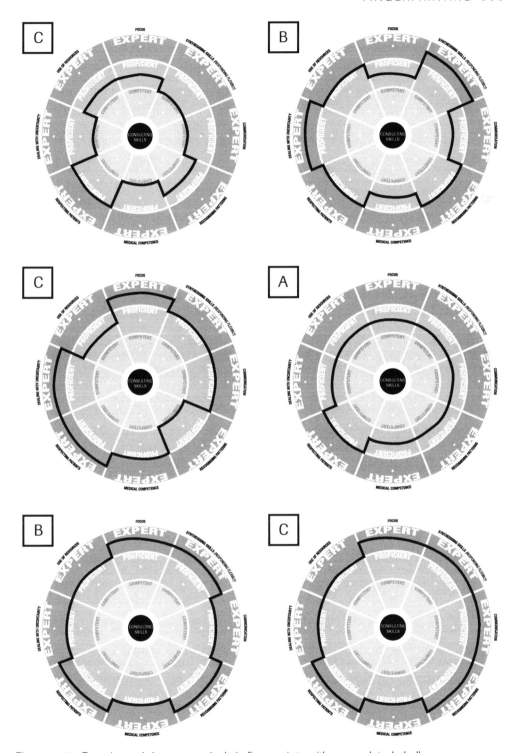

Figure 3.04 Experienced doctor – typical six fingerprints with case related challenge

interpret them slightly differently. Such interpretation should be challenged to aid clarification and assist dialogue.

- The most common marking difficulty arises as a result of identifying indicative statements in more than one performance level, usually over the proficient–expert boundary. There is a temptation to resolve this arithmetically, i.e. if there are more proficient than expert indicators it must be proficient. But some indicators may have more significance than others. The final decision will always involve a judgement, as this is not a 'tick box' kind of Model, but decide on which indicators should have more weighting to the consultation observed. The best fit line on the Impression Graph may tip the judgemental balance. Decide what the key indicators in the consultation were – how appropriate were they?

- Such dilemmas provide useful starting points for feedback: 'I had real difficulty making a decision about . . .'

- The term Synthesising Skills seems to be difficult to grasp, but in the research project, unexpectedly, it was this domain that rated the highest level of marker agreement. It will be seen from the indicative statements that synthesising, 'putting things together', incorporates profound operating qualities such as the level of doctor–patient engagement and the degree of doctor self-awareness. If the consultation is mechanistic and incomplete, there will not be much to synthesise. Summaries shared between doctor and patient provide a useful synthesising indicator.

- Spotting intuitive behaviour is difficult for new doctors, who may not have the experience or language to see what is going on in a fluent consultation. A fluent consultation may be an indicator of intuitive/tacit consulting behaviour. Look for *fluency* and *proactivity* within the consultation in relation to the degree of positive consultation outcomes.

- The label Medical Competence is often interpreted initially as meaning clinical knowledge and skill – understandably. But this domain is concerned with the application of knowledge and skill observable at higher performance levels because the doctor's clinical thinking is shared with the patient.

- Distinguishing between Communication and Respecting Patients sometimes causes trouble, as functioning with high levels of patient respect clearly requires sophisticated communication skills. A useful handhold for this dilemma is to think of communication as eliciting and responding to, as distinct from respecting patients, which is more about shaping the consultation.

GIVING FEEDBACK USING THE CONSULTATION EXPERTISE MODEL

Revisiting the need for feedback

> *'Feedback of one bit or another is essential to all skill acquisition. One cannot improve unless one has ways of judging how good present performance is, and in which direction change must occur.'*[3]

Feedback provides the external input to the internal process of reflection: the affirmation, confirmation and challenge that keeps the learning loop revolving.

Feedback takes time, as does reflection, but time must necessarily be set aside if expertise is to develop. Schön[4] has provided us with the language for professional reflection, key to our notion of expertise development:

- reflecting in action (thinking whilst consulting)
- reflection on action (looking back at what was done)
- willing suspension of disbelief, which allows the learner to try out ideas gained from discussion of the first two without necessarily believing they can succeed.

Feedback enhances the second and third of these by opening up reflection and thus providing ideas to try out in similar circumstances in the future. Fingerprint observations provide the data for feedback.

Giving feedback

Before considering how and what to feedback using the Model, we think it worthwhile to revisit general feedback recommendations.

There are a variety of feedback process models specific to medical education, such as Pendleton's rules[5] or the agenda-led approach (ALOBA).[6] However, it has been found that most experienced practitioners want to cut through the politesse and get down to straight talk. Given the general feedback rules over the page, we have found the critical friend approach, based as it is on professional critique, fits well with the Consultation Expertise Model, as there is sufficient structure in the Model itself either to follow a colleague's expressed needs or provide an agreed sequence of observation.

> *'A critical friend, as the name suggests, is a trusted person who asks provocative questions, provides data to be examined through another lens and offers critique of a person's work as a friend.'*[7]

> *'The task of the critic is to adumbrate, suggest, imply, connote, render, rather than attempt to translate. In this task, metaphor and analogy, suggestion and*

*implication are major tools. The language of criticism, indeed, its success as criticism, is measured by the brightness of its illumination. **The task of the critic is to help us to see.***'[8] [emphasis added]

Experience has shown us that feedback without challenge may limit personal growth and lead to resentment. Challenge, however, must be accompanied by support if feedback is to be constructive, perceived to be useful and lead to a change in behaviour.

FEEDBACK – RULES OF THE GAME

- ❏ Focus on **observed behaviour**, not the person.
- ❏ Focus on **what is seen** – check inferences.
- ❏ Focus on **description rather than judgement**.
- ❏ Focus on specific behaviours within the context in which they occur.
- ❏ Share ideas and information rather than advice.
- ❏ Explore alternatives rather than answers.

Using the Model

As with all feedback, both you and the consulter need to feel relaxed in the awareness that the process is confidential. The consulter may utilise the feedback as evidence within their personal development folder, but this will be their choice.

Where possible, it is best to have fingerprints from several cases in order to discuss an aggregated feedback and thus avoid the possibility of one apparently less-good consultation colouring the whole discussion. This doesn't mean the questionable consultation can't be touched upon, but it need not dominate input into the feedback process.

Whatever structure of feedback is agreed on, the process should be geared to the learner's agenda. It should be based on what is observed in the consultation, and any assumptions or interpretations should be clarified before entering into the discussion proper. For instance, it is easy to assume things have been missed when the consulter has deliberately not 'gone there'. This should be evident from the Fingerprint Case Sheet. In practice we have found that consulters new to the Model seldom have an agenda and that the doctor familiar with the Model leads the initial discussions. With prolonged use of the Model, consulters may wish to choose a particular area of consulting to concentrate on.

In the absence of a specific needs agenda, we have found it useful to start the discussion with the Impression Graph markings to assist with agreeing the consultation performance level for that case.

The Impression Graph allows consideration of the 'fluency' of a particular consultation. Fluency does not necessarily equate to a quicker consultation, as a large part of the fluency is provided by the consulter intuitively following the patient's lead within the consultation. Did the consultation demonstrate 'going there' and how far did it go? How strategic was the management plan? These are good starting points when considering feedback in terms of overall 'expertise' and, of course, as a platform for discussion of consulting skills development as a whole.

Once the Impression Graph has been considered, it's time to move on to the eight domains, where, even with experienced practitioners who weren't overly keen on a Pendleton approach, we've found that first taking the areas where affirmation is easy helps settle colleagues into the substance of the Model. Even such positive areas will involve suggestions for improvement, so it sets the tone before looking at areas where there is more room for development. To assist this, the Feedback Sheets illustrated in the Feedback Pack (*see* Appendix 4) are set out in terms of 'observed behaviours' and 'areas for development'.

Initially, when describing observed behaviours, it is important to include examples of phrases and responses used both by the consulter and the patient. Use terms like 'I saw you do . . .', 'I noticed you said . . .' and 'The patient said . . .' With these observations as a foundation, move on to open discussion about possible alternative behaviours or areas for development. Enabling the consulter to identify with specific examples is advantageous, as it provides a firm basis for discussion and critique.

Throughout the feedback, maintain an open dialogue with the consulter in order to maximise their learning from the process.

Do not be afraid to give more challenging feedback, particularly when colleagues have identified their feedback focus. It is our experience that consulters are often aware of developmental areas and are pleased to have the opportunity to discuss openly options for improvement. This is particularly useful if colleagues feel the fingerprinted consultations represent their usual work.

Having addressed all the appropriate categories, conclude by summarising the discussion with specific reference to items that may be worth including in the personal development plan (PDP). Actual entries in the PDP require a period of consideration if they are to reflect a serious developmental purpose.

Interestingly, we do find it harder to provide constructive developmental suggestions to those who already consult at a high expertise level. Although it can be argued that these doctors are already at a consulting skill pinnacle, it is important to bear in mind that circumstances change and we need to hone skills repeatedly. It is important to think developmentally for everyone.

And finally

It's important to get feedback on the quality of the feedback. There is an art and skill in giving feedback. Does this ring true for the consulter? Has the colleague a clear idea of what to do next? Has the learner's agenda been met? The person giving the feedback needs to hone her or his skills as well!

Feedback responses from the Margaret Henderson research project

I felt I addressed the patient's ideas, concerns and expectation but had not thought of considering my own ICE as the consulter.

I am now looking into seeing things in a wider context.

In summary, I accept that this was a business-like consultation but would like to have displayed more breadth and depth. I will video a few of my consultations and look at how I work with cues and clues.

The feedback was a fair reflection of the skills I demonstrated in the consultation. It was doctor-oriented and I controlled it, probably deliberately. I did not go into the social and psychological side, I think for two reasons. Firstly, it was the first time I saw this patient and chances are she would be seen again with such a chronic problem (backache) and it would have doubled the length of the consultation. The learning point is not to do this – the patient may not come back but rather see someone else. Negotiate more with the patient, even though I will lose control of the consultation, its outcome and the time taken.

FEEDBACK EXAMPLE: THE CASE OF MRS JUDITH ANDERSON

Judith Anderson was developed as a simulation from a recording of a real patient seen by a colleague. As will be gathered from the abbreviated case notes below, Mrs Anderson presents with a complex set of symptoms. In the first instance, Mrs Anderson was taken to the surgeries of all eight doctors in the project team in order to explore the nature of expertise in use with a really challenging patient. Later she was seen by family doctor trainees in their last six months of training to see how they managed such a difficult case (*see* Consultation 1 below).

Subsequently, another colleague, a very experienced practitioner (*see* Consultation 2 below), volunteered to see Mrs Anderson in order to demonstrate the process of recording, fingerprinting and giving feedback. In this case the colleague was asked to provide a recorded case narrative immediately after the consultation to explore another way in which the Model can be used. This has enabled us to illustrate two feedback approaches using the same consultation.

Case notes – Mrs Judith Anderson

Patient Number: 1526	
Personal Details	
Sex	F
Surname	Anderson
Forename	Judith
Date of Birth	63 yrs
Title	Mrs
Marital Status	Married
Medical Record	
Significant problems	
40 yrs ago	Depression 'hysteria' Rx Nardil and LSD therapy
33 yr ago	'Panic attacks' Rx Surmontil and Valium
31 yr ago	Normal pregnancy
29 yr ago	Normal pregnancy
16 yr ago	Barium enema
7 yr ago	# NOF
3 yr ago	Allergic rhinitis
3 yr ago	Bone densiometry hip 93% spine 101%
2 yr ago	TAH BSO ovarian cyst – stage 1 poorly differentiated endometroid carcinoma of ovary
2 yr ago	MRI normal spine
2 yr ago	Neurology referral
Surgery entries	
3 yr ago	Reflux oesophagitis
2.5 yr ago	Flattened affect, small writing? Parkinsons Rx Madopar No help . . . . Neurology
2 yr ago	Neurology referral Rx ropinirole

(continued)

22 m ago	Right frozen shoulder injected
21 m ago	Burning sensation on swallowing Rx Mucaine
18 m ago	Stopped cabergoline because of side effects – very low and agitated – 'help me'. Change Surmontil to paroxetine
19 m ago	RIF pains PR NAD
18 m ago	Migraines Rx Imigran
17 m ago	Doing much better. Less agitated. Read s/e profile of lansoprazole (?hair loss)
14 m ago	Vulvovaginitis Rx Vagifem
11 m ago	Trying to reduce diazepam 6 x 2 mg at present
6 m ago	Down to 4 diazepam per day
5 m ago	Doesn't want to try amantadine as recommended by neuro
4 m ago	Dyspepsia – doesn't want endoscopy
1 m ago	On 5 diazepam. Can't cut food or do buttons up

Referrals

2 yr ago	Neurology referral

Medication

Current Date Commenced	Drug Detail
14 m ago	Vagifem pessaries

Past Date Commenced	Drug Detail
18 m ago	Paroxetine
18 m ago	Imigram
18 m ago	Cabergoline (Neuro)
21 m ago	Mucaine
2 yr ago	Ropinirole (Neuro)
3 yr ago	Surmontil 25 mg tds. Diazepam 2 mg

3 yr ago	Lansoprazole
33 yr ago	Surmontil
40 yr ago	Nardil

As can be seen, Mrs Anderson has a long and complicated history. The case notes (selected and anonymised from the original patient's) also include four letters from the consultant neurologist and two from the specialist registrar in obstetrics and gynaecology not included here but seen by the doctor. Mrs Anderson presents holding a card torn from a Nexium packet but having forgotten why she made the appointment.

Consultation 1 – an experienced trainee
Judith Anderson – a written feedback comparison from a member of the project team in response to a recorded consultation by an experienced trainee.

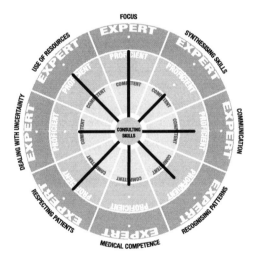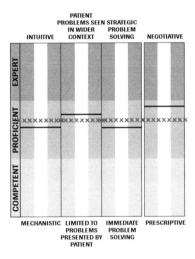

Figure 3.05 Judith Anderson: experienced family doctor specialist registrar – fingerprint and Impression Graph

Overall comment
This was a clearly competent consultation, with the patient's expressed problems being firstly discovered and then managed. The final summary helped to clarify the problems and the plans for both the doctor and the patient.

Impression Graph
Intuitive/mechanistic

There was evidence of intuitive work in the early part of the consultation in persuading the patient to develop her agenda from her initial presentation of not knowing why she'd come. Later in the consultation questions such as 'Is he (patient's husband) being supportive' suggested that you were aware of another aspect to that being presented.

Repeated return to and reliance on the hospital letters made a lot of the actions more mechanistic. Following the cues presented about her husband and family may have led to a more complete assessment and plan.

Problems seen in a wider context

You concentrated on the problems as presented by the patient very well but it was late in the consultation (at about 13 minutes) before you asked about home circumstances and later still before you found out about the patient's children.

It would be interesting to try to see how patients' problems affect their lives and those around them to help develop a comprehensive management plan.

Strategic problem solving

You planned a home visit by the OT, which was a practical idea showing a good use of resources, as well as giving the patient a clear idea of what else you would do.

This did not go beyond the month's follow-up appointment and there was no evidence of what might be done if there were problems with the latest medication.

Negotiation/prescription

During your summary you checked with the patient about her understanding of her problems and the plans and she was happy with them as evidenced by her saying 'I'm happy with that' a couple of times. You were happy to agree to the patient's desire to reduce her Nexium.

There was only a little evidence of negotiation in this plan though, mainly around the patient asking if she could stop the new medication if it didn't suit and whether she could return before the month.

Asking for ideas, concerns and expectations can help to develop negotiation, and this in turn helps with concordance. This case is more difficult than some in that the patient is unclear about what's wrong, so this needs to be done carefully to ensure the patient understands the options she has.

Fingerprint
Communication

At the start of the consultation you didn't interrupt the patient and allowed her to set the scene by not asking anything until nearly a minute had passed and she'd asked you a question. Given that lots of consultations are interrupted by the doctor earlier than this and before the patient has finished what they want to say, this was excellent.

Summarising the consultation was also a very useful tool.

As identified above, you did respond to verbal cues but I couldn't see evidence of your response to her demeanour and I think this may have helped in interpreting some of the non-verbal cues.

Recognising Patterns

You recognised that the patient's initial symptoms suggested Parkinson's disease and proceeded to manage the problem along these lines. You also enquired briefly about depression but didn't follow this up in enough detail to check this as a possibility, even though the patient was on anti-depressants.

The return to the hospital letters suggested uncertainty and an amount of lack of faith in your own judgement.

Medical Competence

Whilst you covered the patient's agenda and also tried to reduce her use of benzodiazepines, you didn't explicitly check her risk of self-harm or suicide, despite her repeated messages that she did not wish to be resuscitated. The single question 'You don't feel like doing away with yourself?' has the problems of being quite direct and also being a negative question inviting the patient to comfort the doctor with 'no' but not necessarily meaning it. Try to use a different approach to this issue, such as 'A lot of people who have complicated problems like yours have thoughts of harming themselves or even killing themselves. These thoughts can be quite frightening, do you get those kinds of thoughts?' or 'You've mentioned not being resuscitated a few times today. I wonder if you ever get thoughts that you'd be better off dead in your current situation.'

Respecting Patients

Your introduction and allowing the patient to express her reasons for attendance were good examples of respect for the patient. You went on to validate her problems as she presented them.

A greater knowledge of her life situation would have developed this further, and trying not to make notes whilst listening to the patient would also help. If you need to make notes in a complex consultation such as this, then an explicit indication that that's what you are doing will aid the patient feeling respected and not make them feel ignored.

Dealing with Uncertainty

There was a lot of uncertainty in this consultation and you were able to help the patient to be clearer about why she had made the appointment and what the next plans were. This was helped by the early listening and the summary.

When challenged by the patient as to what was wrong, you acknowledged the difficulty of not knowing what was wrong with her but didn't pursue this. Instead you returned to the hospital letters.

The use of amantadine, suggested by the hospital, could have been put into greater relief by showing your uncertainty about its efficacy. The offer of a review at a month, or sooner if the patient was troubled, helped this issue.

Use of Resources

The deployment of the OT was a good way of helping this patient and her husband deal with her problems. Checking whether a scan would be useful was also helpful without committing yourself to actually organising an expensive investigation if it was not appropriate.

The consultation was a long one (approx 30 minutes) but this may have been time well spent, as a clear trust in you was being developed by the patient.

Use of Ideas, Concerns and Expectations and a more in-depth view of the effect of the patient's problems on her life and those around her (and of her life and those around her on her problems) may have clarified the management but could be deferred to the next consultation.

Focus

You showed that you had retained focus on a complex presentation by your careful summary. You had recognised the need for a deeper understanding of the patient's problems by offering the OT visit.

This use of summarising is a useful and effective tool in complex consultations.

Whilst you responded to cues about her desire not to be resuscitated and about her husband, this was only after she had made the comments a few times.

Synthesising Skills

This area of the fingerprint is difficult to assess fully on only one consultation but you did identify the presenting problems and dealt with them in turn.

If you look at the patient within their environment earlier in the consultation this may give a wider understanding of their needs and make the management more negotiated rather than prescribed.

Consultation 2 – an experienced practitioner

THE FINGERPRINT CASE SHEET – COMPLETED BY AN
EXPERIENCED DOCTOR AFTER THE CONSULTATION

Reasons for attendance   To discuss reducing dose of Nexium –
also wants to know 'What is wrong'.

Patient's previous events   As per notes   Ix Parkinson's →
non-responsive
Neurologist →
'General System
Decline'

Doctor's previous contacts   N/A

What affected you most in the consultation (thoughts and feelings)

❏   Patient expresses 'powerlessness'
❏   Unhappy marriage – 'trapped'
❏   Life very constrained ??? by disability
❏   More likely now organic

Challenge Rating   C (Confirmed by Responding Doctor)

Colleague doctor's comments on Impression Graph and fingerprint domains using Feedback Sheets from the Fingerprint Pack

Impression Graph

* Intuitive/mechanistic

Willing to allow changes of direction from patient.

* Problems seen in a wider context

Opens up discussion on role of relationship with husband.

* Problems seen in a wider context

Offers broad approach to problem.

* Negotiation/Prescription

Negotiated a lot of areas of problem management.

* Comments

A fluid consultation which covered a lot of issues.

Fingerprint

* Communication

Quiet and calm approach with a lot of clarifying, e.g. 'What made you think of rheumatism?' together with regular summarising.

● Recognising patterns

Depression – impact of relationships noted.

● Respecting patients

All patient's ideas were accepted and accommodated.

● Dealing with uncertainty

*Uncertainty of problem recognised and openly discussed – 'I wouldn't pin your hopes on a single assessment' is an example. [**Comment** – Not necessarily discussed with patient, e.g. pros/cons of therapy]*

● Use of resources

Sensible options offered for problems. Consultation was long; perhaps a little less repetition would have been OK.

● Focus

Able to move with the patient from problem to problem but kept an eye on the overall pattern.

● Synthesising skills

*Used affect as a diagnostic tool – responded to patient with a quiet style [**Comment** – A difficult area to analyse on a single consultation]*

● Comment

All areas were covered at what was clearly an expert level in a case that was difficult and time-consuming.

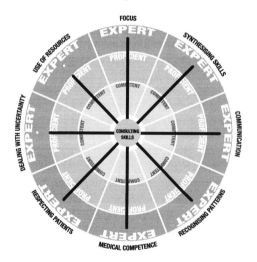 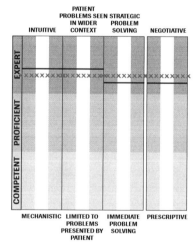

Figure 3.06 Judith Anderson: experienced family doctor – fingerprint and Impression Graph

FEEDBACK – USING A CASE NARRATIVE
CASE NARRATIVE RECORDED BY EXPERIENCED DOCTOR AFTER THE CONSULTATION

I have just seen Judith Anderson, who is a 63-year-old lady, who came in, sat down and first explained that she had forgotten what she had come for. We really explored a number of issues, eventually dealing with the one she had come for, because she remembered about half-way through the consultation. Just to clear that out of the way, she actually came to talk about reducing the dose of Nexium which she is on for her reflux oesophagitis and I agreed to that.

The underlying problem is one of general disability, inability to walk properly, trouble with stairs, difficulty doing buttons, unable to cut up food. In other words she appears as if she has a physical disability of the Parkinsonian type. She has, however, seen the specialist and has been treated with Parkinson's drugs to absolutely no avail. Reading the letter it would appear that the neurologist thinks she has a general, if you like, systems decline but apparently hadn't yet done a brain scan from the notes and the patient seemed sure that she hadn't had one so she is probably correct. I was struck by a number of aspects of the patient's affect. She speaks with a quiet voice, almost timidly. She seems resigned to her state, although she wants to know what it is that is causing the problem. And at various points during the consultation it becomes apparent that she really is trapped in a very unhappy life, in that she has no friends, very little opportunity to get out of the house, that her husband who is retired and extensively cares for her in an outwardly satisfactory fashion will not take her out with him and says, 'oh no you are not fit to do this or that'.

She comes across almost like a caged bird who is sitting there and is unable to find a way out. My thoughts during the consultation were that I wondered if her disability was actually a way of avoiding having to face the possibility that she could leave. She expressed the fact that she would like to leave her husband and take her half and just go but she hasn't the courage to do that. Her disabilities increased around the time that her husband retired. In other words, the more he is around, the more the more disabled she becomes. I think it would be quite interesting to hear the other side of the story, because it is just possible that there is a 'folie a deux' here, where the husband needs her to be disabled and she fulfils that role and is trapped in it but is unhappy in it. However, he may not be like that and this may be a one-sided thing where there have been long-standing relationship difficulties within the marriage, and that has manifested itself in her depression over some 40 years. But at the same time she hasn't got the courage and the strength to face leaving the marriage so the disability provides a very good way of remaining being looked after by her husband and retaining the security of the marriage and home that she has got but without completely giving up the dream of if she was well she would be able to leave.

I think that the way forward is probably for her to have some therapy. It would need to be a therapist of considerable skill and insight. I think she could potentially make some progress with it, but I suppose my dilemma is that we may, if you like, open the cage and she is unable to fly out and she may be no better off. She might be more unhappy if she increases her insight and finds that she hasn't got the courage to leave. So there is just a slight reservation on my part about pursuing the treatment.

She is a very interesting person to meet and talk to and one that I would enjoy looking after as a family doctor because I think the potential to try and unravel some of the difficulties is there if she is able to look at it. Having said that, I realise that if she is unable to move forward she could become something of a long-term problem; a little bit of an effort to look after in the longer term.

COLLEAGUE DOCTOR'S COMMENTS ON THE CASE NARRATIVE USING THE CONSULTATION EXPERTISE MODEL AS A REFERENCE

Colleague doctor: *The immediate thing that I realised from the narrative is that you go beyond the patient's presenting problem and also beyond the purely physical aspects of the case to look at the social and psychological aspects.*

Doctor: *My thoughts during the consultation were that I wondered if her disability was actually a way of avoiding having to face the possibility that she could leave. She expressed the fact that she would like to leave her husband and take her half and just go but she hasn't the courage to do that. Her disabilities increased around the time that her husband retired. In other words the more he is around the more disabled she becomes.*

In terms of the Model this might be seen as the interaction being used for therapeutic as well as diagnostic means (Synthesising Skills expert-level descriptor).

Colleague doctor: *To do this you used not only the verbal but also the non-verbal aspects of her presentation: 'I was struck by a number of aspects of the patient's affect. She speaks with a quiet voice, almost timidly, she seems resigned to her state although she wants to know what it is that is causing the problem.' (Synthesising Skills expert descriptor level, uses affect of the patient as a diagnostic tool.) This was borne out by seeing the consultation on tape later.*

You are clearly able to manage complex issues, recognising that the patient had to have time to remember her reason for coming and dealing with that alongside the complex psychology of the case. (Recognising Patterns, Medical Competence, Synthesising Skills.)

An awareness of the uncertainties in this case comes from the potential difficulties you saw in helping the patient to 'escape' her situation.

Doctor: *She might be more unhappy if she increases her insight and finds that she hasn't got the courage to leave. So there is just a slight reservation on my part about pursuing the treatment.*

Colleague doctor: *This is interesting, as in the fingerprinting I didn't feel I'd seen much use of uncertainty and so had marked this aspect at the borderline of proficient and expert. The only other area I marked as on this border was Use of Resources and this was based on the timing of the consultation. There was some repetition of aspects of the consultation and I wondered if it could have been shorter. This is a minor criticism as this is a complex case and wasn't an issue picked up in your narrative.*

EXPERIENCED DOCTOR'S REFLECTION ON THE FEEDBACK AND FINGERPRINTING PROCESS

This is based on my first experience of the fingerprinting process.

The face-to-face feedback was fairly brief, and I think part of that was the fact that most of it was in the expert level of assessment. I appreciate that it is easier to have a learning dialogue when there are definite areas of potential change and improvement. That is not to say I don't have things to learn, but I think the only way to do it would be to go through the tape and pick out points together.

For me, and for the future, it was lack of immediacy that reduced the impact – perhaps not helped by the time lag between the consultation and the feedback because of squeezing the feedback into busy schedules as an 'extra'. If it were compulsory for reaccreditation, for example, time for the consultation and the feedback would have to be prioritised.

Maybe fingerprinting and feedback has to be done as a package – e.g. consultation one week, and feedback session the following week. In terms of cost-effectiveness, it would make sense to cover the practice as a unit with a series of consultations for the different partners one half day, followed by individual or even joint feedback as a group the following week – it would be really interesting to be part of such a project.

References

1. Broadfoot P. Assessment and intuition. In: Atkinson T, Claxton G. *The Intuitive Practitioner.* Buckingham: Open University Press; 2000. p. 200.
2. Dreyfus H, Dreyfus S. *Mind over Machine: the power of human intuition and expertise in the era of the computer.* New York: Free Press; 1986. p. 27.

3. Slobada J. Acquiring skill. In: Gellatly A, editor. *The Skilful Mind: an introduction to cognitive psychology.* Milton Keynes: Open University Press; 1986. p. 33.

4. Schön D. *Educating the Reflective Practitioner.* San Francisco: Jossey-Bass;1987.

5. Pendleton D, Schofield T, Tate P, *et al. The New Consultation: developing doctor-patient communication.* Oxford: Oxford University Press; 2003. pp. 75–80.

6. Kurtz S, Silverman J, Draper J. *Teaching and Learning Communication Skills in Medicine.* Oxford: Radcliffe Medical Press; 1998.

7. Costa L, Kallick A. Through the Lens of a Critical Friend. *Educ Leadersh.* 1993; **51**(2): 49–51.

8. Eisner E. *The Art of Educational Evaluation.* London: Falmer Press; 1985. pp. 147–61.

4   USES OF THE MODEL

The facility to fingerprint consultations extends use of the Model beyond the original purpose of providing doctors in training with a picture of how their consulting expertise might develop. The Model and fingerprinting have been used by colleagues in a variety of ways:
- for appraisal and revalidation portfolios
- by practising doctors
  - for personal reflection
  - for exchange between colleagues
- by family doctor trainers with family doctor specialist registrars
- by programme directors and doctor trainer groups
- as part of an expertise-development teaching programme.

Other unexplored but potential uses are:
- for whole practice training
- for performance tracking and change with remediation.

What follows will provide a picture of several ways in which the Model has been or can be used. However, first a few helpful tips we've learned from introducing the Model to groups of advisers, trainers, practising family doctors and postgraduate specialist registrars that are worth sharing.

INTRODUCING THE CONSULTATION EXPERTISE MODEL TO COLLEAGUES
Practising doctors can pick up a Fingerprint Pack and have a go at fingerprinting a consultation and so become familiar with the Model simply by using it. However, many users may prefer to achieve some prior understanding by means of an introduction from someone already familiar with the Model. So far this has been done on a one-to-one basis with busy doctors over a lunch break, with a practice team at a CPD meeting or protected learning event and more formally as a workshop with practising doctors, trainers and specialist registrars.

The Model needs careful introduction

At first sight the Model can appear daunting, so we have explored how best to explain it. Experience has shown it necessary to communicate the basic structure of the Model first.

1.   Explain the four components of the circular model:
     — the consulting skill core
     — the three performance levels
     — the eight domains
     — the indicative statements.

For this we generally use a PowerPoint presentation because it can be used with a few colleagues around a laptop or through a projector.

2.   Compare a videotaped extract of consultations with the same simulated patient by a new and a very experienced doctor. This enables us to hone in on the nature of higher-order expertise. It becomes apparent, for example, that the experienced doctor's approach is proactive rather than reactive; a big difference, but one dependent on experience.
3.   Whatever the size of group, we do a fingerprinting exercise using a volunteered consultation recording. Coping with all eight domains to start with can be off-putting, so we ask people to concentrate on marking one or two domains only as a contribution to a composite group fingerprint, i.e. a fingerprint put together from a number of contributors. This works particularly well with larger groups split into fingerprinting teams of eight. Group fingerprints can then be compared, and of course the process can be illustrated quickly by this means.

These three activities can provide the structure for an introductory programme:
● the four components of the Model
● an illustration of advanced consulting
● how to fingerprint.

It is, however, the detailed insights and understandings explored within such a structure that are essential to appreciate how the Model may be used and, more importantly, whether to adopt it.

Explain the connection between expertise development and experience

It is probably self-evident to initiates that growth in expertise is dependent upon experience. What is not so evident is that experience in itself is not sufficient. Indeed, years of experience may lead to little or no change in expertise. For all but the few effortless self-learners, changes in expertise need reflection and deliberation. It is necessary to elaborate this point because the Model provides one objective means whereby learning from experience can be assisted. The need for reflection time will not be new to most doctors. Nevertheless, it is worth a reminder.

The idea that the Model is predicated on experience over time is a crucially important point because new family doctors need to appreciate that their fingerprints will rarely extend into the expert outer circle until they have longer experience – experience cannot be fast-tracked. There is no point in new family doctors becoming disheartened because their fingerprints only fall within the competent or proficient levels. With this in mind, the educational purpose of introducing the Model to doctors with limited experience needs to be considered carefully. **We suggest the educational purpose lies in providing new doctors with a clear idea of how their consulting may change with experience and of the consulting attributes they might aspire to over time.**

The Model exposes the complexity of advanced consulting: this takes time to explain

Early comments that the Model is too complex drove us to a deeper level of thinking. There was a temptation to do a rethink and simplify. But this floundered on what we realised was the unalterable fact that **expert consulting is by its very nature complex**. In retrospect, it is interesting that we came upon this realisation experientially in response to colleagues' reaction before encountering the growing literature on complexity theory. How to explain this and still promote the Model caused us some difficulty.

Despite promotion over many years, it would appear that a patient-centred approach is not deeply embedded in professional practice, particularly at the level of the shared decision making advocated by Elwyn[1] and others.[2,3] Why is this? To speculate, is it possible that family doctors in training are not intellectually prepared for this change of emphasis? To explore the point, doctors leave medical school with clinical method deeply ingrained in their professional behaviour. It is essential; indeed, it is the default mode: history-taking, examination, diagnosis, management – a rational linear process. As such, clinical method is a **complicated** process in the sense that each stage can be isolated and improved in such a way that the overall outcome may be improved – it's scientific and safe.

But what happens if a doctor does engage with the patient's agenda? What the patient says may take the doctor into all kinds of unpredictable arenas. The doctor responds to what the patient says and asks important clinical questions, the answers to which may take the conversation in yet another direction and so on, throughout an interaction that is part doctor agenda, part patient agenda – not a rational linear process. In fact, what happens as soon as a doctor truly attends to the patient socially and affectively is that the thinking process goes from complicated mode, as in clinical method, to **complex** mode, as in a holistic (gestalt) type thinking that is, in part, not predictable; that is affective as much as rational; or, when intuitive, appears to be unscientific. Elsewhere we make the suggestion that it is neither logical nor illogical, it is non-logical.[4]

> 'Describing the consultation as a complex, adaptive system provides a coher-
> ent theoretical basis for understanding the consultation which has so far been
> lacking.'[5]

In this sense expert consulting is complex. It is complex because the doctor is dealing with ever-changing variables. There is a logic to complicated linear thinking, $a+b+c = d$. This is not the case with complex thinking, where meaning has to be sucked out of a series of disconnected variables, often sequentially in a challenging consultation.

Switching to the thinking frame required for family doctoring is what Patricia Benner, in her study of nursing expertise, refers to as a 'qualitative leap or discontinuity in problem approach.'[6] With this leap in mind, we have to accept that while the Consultation Expertise Model may appear to be complex, its complexity has to be confronted simply because higher levels of consulting are complex. Simplification would not be appropriate!

INTRODUCING THE CONSULTATION EXPERTISE MODEL

Two key issues:
1. expertise is predicated on reflective experience acquired over many years
2. family doctor consultations that engage affectively in shared decision making with the patient are by definition complex – dealing with ever-changing unpredictable variables.

USING THE CONSULTATION EXPERTISE MODEL FOR APPRAISAL AND REVALIDATION

As we write this book we know that we are likely as family doctors to have to undergo revalidation. Some of the evidence for this process will be derived from the appraisal process,[7] but as yet we do not know what will be acceptable. Just as certification, for example summative assessment, requires a structured assessment of consultation competence, it is likely that an equivalent assessment will be necessary for revalidation.

You may wish to consider the performance criteria in the RCGP Consultation Observation Tool (COT)[8] and decide how helpful you would find feedback in relation to those criteria for your stage of professional development.

Both COT and the fingerprinting process derived from the Consultation Expertise Model can be used with videotaped consultations, so there is no reason why you should not receive feedback on your videotaped consulting performance using both the COT and the Consultation Expertise Model fingerprinting tool. Remember that fingerprinting depends upon the judgement of peers. If your consultations are being peer-observed directly, it would be impractical to complete assessments using two methods at the same time.

Both assessments will provide evidence for inclusion in an appraisal folder. Bear in mind though that unless you have sufficient experience to be a fluent consulter it may be more difficult to find educational value using Consultation Expertise Model-based fingerprints.

Key to your effective personal use of the Consultation Expertise Model fingerprinting tool is finding the appropriate person to observe the consultation and give you feedback. An observer needs to be able to do the following things:

1. accurately observe what happens in the consultation in relation to the indicative statements
2. reach a consistent judgement about the performance level in each of the domains
3. provide sensitive and appropriate feedback as elaborated in the fingerprinting section.

The evidence in the appraisal folder can be enhanced by completing a reflective sheet following feedback from your colleague.

USE BY A PRACTISING FAMILY DOCTOR – FEEDBACK FROM A COLLEAGUE USING THE CONSULTATION EXPERTISE MODEL FOR SELF-REFLECTION
HOW DID YOU START?

With a lot of procrastination! Getting organised and getting the camera in the room was quite difficult, so it needed a bit of personal nagging and a bit of self-discipline to make it happen. I let the girls at the front desk know. We have a touch screen in the practice, so I had to consent the patients before I saw them as well as after. I had to check that the partners were happy as well. I then just recorded some videos and watched on TV at home. I watched three from morning surgery – then there was a very good one to analyse, so I went for that and I skimmed through the others. The others didn't have that much meat in them. I just fingerprinted the one. I have not been there for long, so I don't have an ongoing relationship with patients who know me. I looked through eight consultations, but I only fingerprinted one.

TO WHAT EXTENT DID YOU FOLLOW THE FINGERPRINT PACK AS A GUIDE?

I didn't. I was printing MRCGP consent forms at home the night before, having adapted them online. But actually the consent forms in the pack are very good! It would have been much easier to use them.

WHY DID YOU CHOOSE THAT CASE?

I am not so sure. There are areas I'm aware I'm not too hot on. Maybe I chose one that fits into such an area instinctively because I am self-reflective. You will miss out on blind spots anyway because nobody else is watching it with you. If I was totally new to fingerprinting, I think I'd want to watch a whole surgery, pick three to four consultations and do all of them to get used to it.

It was the kind of case where I feel I am not able to stay in control. People who come in with multiple problems but who also have an anxiety element. Complex stuff like drug abuse as well. Like a firework consultation – can go about 40 different ways. If I am tired and stressed, I can find myself going down an alley I didn't wanted to go down and I am running late. It is the kind of consultation I find quite difficult.

AND THE CASE?

A chap I had seen before – 36-year-old – dire past history – using a lot of drugs – using cannabis – got a sweating problem – social stuff not very good as well – with him you have a physical symptom that is probably anxiety-related and drug-related, for which there are other physical things that could be contributing to the symptoms he is getting. Uncertainty is an area I always struggle to manage. There is a problem here – managing my own uncertainty and not over-investigating inappropriately. The other thing is – I pick up cues very well – that is one of my skills – when I do that I have to decide which cues I follow up. When I was consulting with him there were certain cues I was ignoring. Actually, watching the recording, I was thinking – was I safe to ignore that? Should I have picked them up? – but actually looking at it I was doing well – had I gone down that alley I would have been 20 minutes down the line not having done much good.

FINGERPRINT CASE SHEET: CLASSIFIED AS B

Reasons for attendance – skin condition – sweaty. Complicated by back pain – cannabis and diazepam use – a complex history

Patient's previous events – newish to practice

Doctor's previous contact – one previous contact – sweaty + back pain

What affected you most in the consultation?
When should I refer him?
How suicidal is he now?
I don't want him on diazepam – but will amitriptyline work?
I don't want him to be dependent – but this is complex.

CAN WE LOOK AT THE TECHNICALITIES? HOW DID YOU FIND THE IMPRESSION GRAPH?

The Impression Graph is good in that it gets you to think more broadly, but I couldn't see myself as expert. I tend to mark myself low anyway. I know I'm competent and that there are some good skills there. I was kind of stuck in the proficient area. There is no way I could have marked myself up. I presumed it would be the same as the fingerprint but it wasn't. With the fingerprint, because you've got the word pictures and descriptions of what you are doing, it's not at all tick boxsy. I thought yes I did do that – I am up here – but because of the indicative statements I have to give myself an expert rating for some areas, which is not naturally what I do.

HOW DID YOU BALANCE MODESTY WITH OBJECTIVITY – IT MUST BE DIFFICULT ON YOUR OWN?

I think modesty does come into it, but on the other hand, because of the statements you can say, I did do that – it happened in the consultation. The indicative statements provided the objectivity and helped me cope with my discomfort with the expert rating – they got round my modesty. I would never give myself an A on other scales but with this you have to. I was particularly concerned with the area of Medical Competence; you have to mark that within the bounds of your own understanding. You may be medically competent but you don't actually know. Even though the marking is about application and sharing medical knowledge with the patient, you may as a part-timer feel less secure in that area. But once again, the word pictures help.

DID YOU GO BACK AND ADJUST THE IMPRESSION GRAPH AS MIGHT HAPPEN IF YOU WERE DISCUSSING THIS WITH A COLLEAGUE WHO'D SEEN THE CONSULTATION?

No, I thought it more honest to leave it like that.

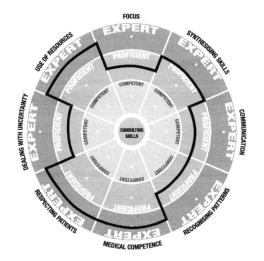 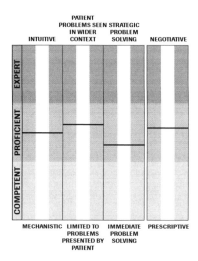

Figure 4.01 Marked fingerprint and Impression Graph

DID YOU USE THE REFLECTION SHEET?

Yes, it was useful. It helped me with what I was thinking and feeling and writing down things I hadn't verbalised before. For example, I did pick up a lot of cues, but I also ignored a lot. But by doing that I increased my uncertainty. If I ignore cues, I think, 'Should I have done this, should I have picked it up'. By picking up cues, by ignoring some, I finish on time. On the other hand, if you 'go there', you have more to contain. With this patient you could be there forever. It's particularly important for somebody else looking at the tape to know this (an example of what might be on the Fingerprint Case Sheet). It was useful for me to verbalise this.

On the surface it was very patient-centred, very negotiative, quite paternalistic. The cues I did ignore I was quite happy about – I did contain it, which is a relief because I feel uneasy when I take risks. I was aware I was picking up cues and storing them – some I go straight into – with one I just smiled and put my eyebrow up in response to his cue and on he went and that was quite intuitive. There was a cue about, *living on his own*, that was slightly flirtatious in nature and straight away I remember thinking, 'I'm not going there'. He sends out mothering need cues, so I have to be aware of transference.

What I really want to do next is record some consultations that don't go so well. Ideally this would mean doing videos on a more regular basis, maybe doing one video surgery every six months. Practically this will be difficult. I like looking at ones which have gone wrong to try and work out why they went wrong. There is a family I'd love to record – they come in with three generations and the consulting room is in chaos. How do you consult with a mother who doesn't speak brilliant English and a kid who speaks relatively good English with all the family dynamic all around you? I really would value a video. The obvious thing to do is to swap and share videos together. We have talked about it at the practice.

RECORDED ON THE REFLECTION SHEET

This is the kind of consultation I find difficult because of:

Complex social dynamics – drug use/abuse – physical problem – medicinal risk/benefit – risk he goes on a bender – 10 minute constraint – possibility of losing control.

I am actually quite 'controlling', although on the surface it all seems patient-centred and negotiated. I was aware of 'ignored' cues to allow me to finish in reasonable time.

A lot of the risk/benefit was not fully negotiated although it was hinted at. Options other than amitriptyline were not discussed because I do not see them as being appropriate at this stage.

I felt pleased with myself, I controlled a consultation which could have gone in a variety of directions and easily become chaotic, mirroring the patient's parallel chaotic lifestyle. As I love going off at tangents and am naturally not very focused, this pleased me.

From the patient's perspective, he wants a magic cure, to move on, to be off cannabis and have a girlfriend. There is no magic cure, but he is moving on – I affirmed that as there are signs he's getting there with the cannabis. One part of me would take him home, adopt him and give him the care I reckon he missed in childhood. As a professional, can I meet him 'adult to adult', give him respect and encouragement, as well as being a good doctor?

In this consultation, for me the problems were: my uncertainty, risk management, deciding which cues to pick up and which to ignore.

Key learning points
- ❏ I pick up a lot of cues and ignore a lot to stay within time.
- ❏ This increases my uncertainty, an area I always find difficult.
- ❏ It makes me take risks, again something I don't do easily.
- ❏ How can I check out if I am right? How can I lessen the stress this involves?

> ## USING THE CONSULTATION EXPERTISE MODEL FOR SELF REFLECTION
>
> **Advice**
> Scan the Fingerprint Pack and remove consent form.
> Tell colleagues what you are doing – record.
> Choose one or more consultations you **want** to review.
> Be sure to complete the Fingerprint Case Sheet.
> View recording(s).
> Reflect using feelings as well as thoughts.
> Disclose and record.

USE BY A FAMILY DOCTOR TRAINER

When the Model was first made public, it was suggested that trainers might find it useful to first select one domain in which it would be timely to extend the quality of a trainee's consulting. The indicative statements within the chosen domain can then be used to provide a statement that may reflect what the trainee is doing and then other indicative statements can be used to discuss what might be done differently.

Given our experience of the conflicting pressures on trainees prior to certification, we tread cautiously. We recommend that use be limited to those postgraduate specialist registrars – ST3 – who have either gained certification prior to the completion of training or who are sufficiently confident in their final months of training to go beyond their comfort zone. We are also wary of using the Model in its entirety before registrars are more generally aware of the context of future expertise growth, as explained above.

Using one domain as a teaching resource at an appropriate moment in a joint surgery or consultation tutorial seems like a good starting point. As with all new approaches, it is equally important for the trainer to feel confident about using the Model. The following narrative, edited from an interview transcript, records how one local trainer employed this approach.

I'd thought about using the Model and needed an opportunity to try it out, needed a suitable registrar who'd be the sort of person who'd find it useful. It turned out that 'A' was that sort of person. We'd done various other consultations in which she did all the right things according to the well-known models. But we still felt there was something missing in her consultations. Something that wasn't quite right, that we couldn't put our finger on. This was a mutual dialogue we'd arrived at from looking at videos. We wanted to find something that would take us a little bit further on.

I had come across the Model but didn't exactly know how to use it. At first, it's a big circle with lots of areas. As we were doing a joint surgery I sat and watched her consult, searching to find some words of wisdom as to how things might improve. I took the Model and the circle and looked at the various definitions as she was consulting. I then focused down on the one area which seemed to be relevant to her kind of consulting. We worked with that segment and forgot about the rest. It was the Focus domain.

I think it was because her consultations were sort of darting around a bit – it's a problem at our practice – we've lots of patients with complex social needs. They come in with one problem and immediately the whole thing branches into about five different problems. Half are socially or financially based and you then throw in the hypertension, obesity, arthritis, the dog dying and everything else. Immediately, you wonder how on earth you can maintain this complex picture and focus it on areas you can work with. That's how we came to Focus – she felt that some of her consultations were not focused. Some of them ended up being a bit woolly and going all over the place. So I used those images and looked at the indicative statements while sitting in the next joint surgery. There was one consultation that fitted the bill. It was a proficient consultation. We looked at shifting the focus between all the different areas and how it could be managed and *how you could try to link them in the patient's mind as well*, so they didn't become independent issues. Sometimes patients themselves hadn't made connections between two areas in their life. Suddenly the light goes on. They realise the two are connected.

The indicative statements were more helpful in trying to do the fingerprinting. My personal difficulty was getting into an appropriate dialogue with 'A'. This Model is about higher-order skills well away from the basics. So you know there isn't one way – there may be 20 or 30 different ways of developing focus in any different number of doctors, so I expect the emphasis is going to be on my skill in using the Model with another doctor. The useful thing was that it gave her a peg to hang it on. Focus isn't a feature in other models. You could do a consultation which was all over the place and still tick boxes – but I felt there was something about this consultation that could be improved. I can still have similar feelings – I've ticked all the right boxes but still haven't quite got to the bottom of a consultation.

It enabled us to identify an aspect of her consulting that didn't feature in other ways of understanding the consultation. It opened up an insight into what was happening in the consultation that could be improved. It showed us what was going on that needed to be worked on. It didn't immediately suggest solutions, but it helped us diagnose the bit she was struggling with. We were able to highlight those areas and talk about them. How do we keep the focus on things? Sometimes letting the focus wander off is quite useful. Sometimes, if you are coming to a bit which the patient is finding very difficult to handle, releasing the focus and going somewhere else is a useful way of relieving pressure and so on.

As you move towards the expert level, the solution-finding is going to get more subtle and more personal – individual for individual doctors. Some of it is experience and some is time – seeing enough patients of that kind and getting your head around it. Recognising the complicated pattern of behaviour the patient has when they walk into the room. You have been there – you immediately pick up how this patient is behaving. 'A' was slightly stilted and she knew that. The bit we looked at was kind of useful as a way of understanding where she was going.

USING THE CONSULTATION EXPERTISE MODEL: POSTGRADUATE TRAINING

Selecting one domain appropriate to immediate trainee development need is recommended for first use of the Model. Such an approach can be useful for:

a. extending the expertise of quick learners who are already competent consulters

b. trainee doctors with a 'blind spot' for whom consideration of a relevant domain with its indicative statements may help unblock stuck behaviour by suggesting alternative strategies.

USE WITH A FAMILY DOCTOR TRAINER GROUP

The group
The group has 10 members. They meet every two or three months to provide mutual support, keep up to date and engage in educational discussion related to training family doctor registrars. Five of the seven members attending this session were familiar with the Model from a previous introductory session. As a consequence, one member requested this further opportunity to fingerprint one of his consultations.

Fingerprinting
Given the length of time since the introductory session, group members did not have sufficient confidence to fingerprint all categories in one go. It was therefore decided to do a composite fingerprint, each member being allocated to one discrete domain and all seven fingerprinting the remaining category: Communication Skills.

The case
An elderly woman presented with a previously known knee problem and said she was 'down in the dumps'. The consultation followed a telephone triage contact. The

doctor examined the knee and discussed previous and ongoing treatment at the hospital. Agreement was reached on this point. Then in response to the unhappy demeanour and 'down in the dumps' cue, a complex emotional story emerged. To start with the woman was caring for her husband, who was suffering from dementia. Of more concern was the fact that the patient's daughter had cut herself off from her mother and never wanted to see her again. The doctor listened to the tearful story in full, how it happened and how, ever since, the patient had cried daily for six months. It was 'like a grieving'. The doctor empathised and suggested practical possibilities such as writing letters even if they were not responded to. Eventually, summarising the low mood and possible depression, the doctor suggested low-dose antidepressants. The patient appeared to agree and a follow-up visit was arranged.

The consultation lasted 24 minutes and was classified, by consensus, as B challenge.

The fingerprint

A composite fingerprint was drawn but not immediately related to the case, because the dialogue focused on the 'dove-hawk' interpretation of expert behaviour. Without going into detail, expert behaviour was identified.

Case feedback discussion

- The contributing doctor was surprised at the fingerprint's high rating because he didn't feel he was challenged by the case.
- The 24 minutes taken was considered to be justified for long-term gain.
- There was much discussion regarding the doctor's decision to deal with the knee problem before the 'down in the dumps' cue. Was the knee the entry ticket and was it connected to the emotional condition? This was not checked out with the patient. There was a subsequent discussion about intuiting patient expectations and the 'connecting' aspect of examining first. The patient wasn't asked!
- As there was a 'lot of listening', the group wanted to know to what extent the doctor was feeling anxious about the extended time taken.
- Most discussion focused on the manner in which the assumption of depression was made and prescribed for without risk assessment and negotiation – a discussion that continued after the end of the session.

Feedback on the Consultation Expertise Model process

- The fingerprinting feedback prompted the question, 'Given the trusting nature of the group, would the above discussion have taken place without the impetus of the Model?' There was agreement that an open case analysis would certainly have followed a straightforward viewing of the consultation but that the Consultation Expertise Model process has additional advantages in:

— prompting an analysis with a common language for neutral feedback
— presenting a structure for the progressive development of consulting expertise
— providing evidence of professional reflection based on publicly known criteria that can be used for appraisal and revalidation.

- There is a possibility that established 'trusting' groups will find it difficult to avoid being lenient and over-marking colleagues. This raises the question of standards, shared standards and the extent to which the indicative statements provide sufficiently strong interpretative guidance.

Post-event feedback – second-level feedback

- Subsequent consideration of this fingerprinting and feedback event gave rise to deeper feedback issues for at least one group member.
- To what extent was the recorded case a therapeutic consultation, given the quality of the doctor's listening and gentle commenting?
- How trustworthy are judgements such as 'she probably expected me to deal with the knee first' and 'from what you have told me you seem to be depressed' (or similar language) if they are not checked with the patient?
- How secure are depression diagnoses without more formal risk management questions?

Comment

The Model can provide an opportunity for a relatively safe group discussion with real depth.

USING THE CONSULTATION EXPERTISE MODEL: DOCTOR TRAINERS

A volunteer prepared to disclose and talk through problems with the group brings a recording of a case that challenged them.

The group has sufficient familiarity with fingerprinting to keep focus on the case rather than the methodology.

Expertise issues should be identified and confronted.

The manner in which personal issues are discussed may determine the future of this process.

References

1. Elwyn G. *Shared Decision Making: patient involvement in clinical practice.* Nijmegan: WOK; 2001.
2. McWhinney R. *A Textbook of Family Medicine.* 2nd ed. New York: Oxford University Press; 1997.
3. Stewart M, Brown JB, Weston WW *et al. Patient-Centered Medicine: transforming the clinical method.* 2nd ed. Oxford: Radcliffe Medical Press; 2003.
4. Sweeney K. *Complexity in Primary Care: understanding its value.* Oxford: Radcliffe Medical Press; 2006.
5. Innes AD, Campion PD, Griffiths FE. Complex consultations and the 'edge of chaos'. *Br J Gen Pract.* 2005; **55**(510): 47–52.
6. Benner P. *From Novice to Expert: excellence and power in clinical nursing practice.* New Jersey: Prentice Hall; 1984. p. 297.
7. www.rcgp.org.uk/default.aspx?page=5635 (accessed 12 August 2008).
8. Can be downloaded from 'resources' section at www.rcgp-curriculum.org.uk/nmrgcp/wpba/consultation_observation_tool.aspx (accessed 12 August 2008).

5 ADVANCED CONSULTING AND THE MODEL: KEY CONCEPTS

KEY CONCEPTS IN RELATION TO 'CONSULTING SKILLS'
Problem framing
What is known

Problem framing is the process by which we attempt to make sense of a patient's presentation. It is concerned with the way information is initially classified or categorised and what happens to this classification when new information appears when time is short. It mainly involves prioritising information – deciding what is relevant and what is not. It is the very individual reasoning pattern which seems to follow the moment of establishing an initial hypothesis – it often involves short-cuts (heuristics) which are inevitably taken to deal with uncertainty under times of pressure.

Short-cuts are techniques for shortening decision making, based on assumptions formed from knowledge or past experience. They always involve an element of risk-taking but are often a valid, reliable and necessary way to make decisions based on limited information, i.e. 'safe risks'. By searching through specific pockets of information to limit the range of possible explanations, short-cuts allow possible solutions to be generated more quickly and effectively. They can be dangerous, however, when based on insufficient relevant knowledge or invalid assumptions.

Common short-cuts and biases
- Confirmatory bias
  - Interpreting new information as being consistent with a favoured hypothesis and ignoring new information inconsistent with a favoured hypothesis.
- Regret bias
  - Overestimation of probability of more serious but treatable diseases, because doctor would hate to miss one.
- Representativeness ('pattern recognition')
  - When a new presentation appears similar to previous case(s) or a known diagnostic category, the tendency to assume that this new presentation is 'representative' and perhaps requiring less vigorous analysis.

- Order effect
  - Information presented early in a consultation (primacy) or late (recency) given greater weight than justified.
- Conservatism
  - 'Anchoring' one's thinking to the first hypothesis and making overly cautious 'adjustments' in the face of new information.
- Attributions
  - The influence of personal biases in interpreting patient presentations (e.g. 'women are more prone to psychological distress', 'drug takers bring medical problems on themselves').

Whereas empathic skill is concerned with identifying dominant clues to the patient's thoughts and feelings about the problem, problem framing skill is concerned with identifying dominant clues to the problem as you see it, i.e. identifying your frame.

KEY STATEMENTS TAKEN FROM A WORKSHOP ON PROBLEM FRAMING, LEICESTER 2004, BY TIM NORFOLK, INSTITUTE OF WORK PSYCHOLOGY, SHEFFIELD UNIVERSITY

- ❏ It takes longer to build the relevant knowledge base than it does to challenge your assumptions.
- ❏ The more 'networks' of knowledge or experience you have access to, the greater the chance of finding a valid solution. Expert family doctors narrow the range of options by searching through illness 'scripts' or 'patterns' for a match with the limited information presented by the patient.
- ❏ The challenge in order to become an expert family doctor is to be able to prioritise information from more diverse networks of medical knowledge and experience whilst also developing safe short-cuts to help speed up the process.
- ❏ The early stages of problem framing largely involve internal reasoning, based on the immediate patient presentation and connections between this and the doctor's personal knowledge and experience. The latter stages of problem framing should actively involve the patient.
- ❏ Because there is no 'gold standard' style for problem framing to model, the focus for individuals wishing to develop further is on recognising their own emergent problem framing style – both in terms of strengths and developmental areas.

Interpersonal skills

> *'Lest we forget, for countless patients it is the telling of their stories that helps to make them well.'*[1]

Interpersonal skills are usually thought of as a taken-for-granted sub-set of communication skills, within which, as experience accrues, is an increasingly influential perceptiveness about people in general. We have stated in the main text that interpersonal skills not only develop in parallel with clinical expertise but, in an extended form, provide the means whereby clinical skills can be applied expertly in family medicine. It is necessary to unpack this further if we are to assist the expertise journey.

What's the problem?

During training the focus is on levels of interpersonal skill appropriate for certification and subsequently, in the Dreyfus sense, on competent consulting. There is little consideration of skill progression over time. As a consequence, what constitutes an advanced interpersonal skill is left undefined.

This latter point creates problems for expertise development post-certification. Colleagues or teachers are left with an **undeveloped interpersonal skill language**. For example, an observer might say, 'You left some productive silences.' But why were they productive? There are many contributing factors to a 'productive' silence – eye messages, invitational voice tone, maybe an echo question here, a shift in listening mode there and so on – as Glyn Elwyn puts it, the 'gaze on the micro-communication processes within inter-personal interactions'.[2]

There can even be **confusion over what constitutes an interpersonal skill**. Finding out why the patient has come is often regarded as a communication skill whereas it is actually a clinical task requiring questioning and other interpersonal skills.

Interpersonal skill language for expertise development

It is important to clarify the difference between skills and skilled behaviours in order that we can provide observational feedback in a shared language. Interpersonal skills are analytically singular and are thus easy to identify for feedback. For example, questioning is a skill that can be divided into sub-skills such as open, closed, circular or echo questions, whereas skilled interpersonal behaviours, such as establishing rapport or eliciting disclosure, are composite skills. They are dependent on the use of singular skills. Rapport, for example, may be achieved by demeanour or tone of voice or alternatively, by assertive straight talking; whatever skills suit the context. It is skilled behaviours that are context-specific to family medicine. Reassurance would be a case in point – always related to a clinical situation.

It is important to distinguish between medically skilled behaviour and the interpersonal skills that underpin them.

Progression in interpersonal skill and skilled behaviour development

'For behaviour to be regarded as skilled, it must be learned.'[3]

Skilled behaviours by implication develop or decline in their application over time. If, according to Hargie above, they can be learned, we need to know what is to be learned. Unfortunately, this is relatively unexplored territory, so we must conjecture what is likely to happen as expertise develops. The diagrams below outline possible progression based on practitioner experience and observation of consultation video-tapes from experienced doctors covering a wide variety of patient conditions.

'When patients feel their cues have been acknowledged, they will speed up their disclosure rate, and this will make the interview more efficient and effective.'[4]

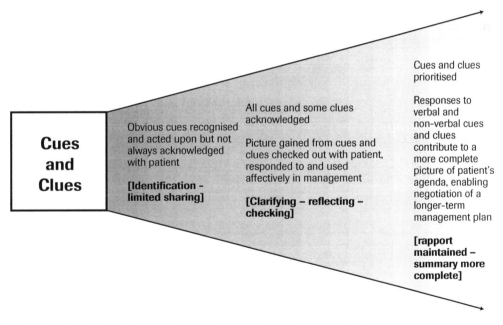

Figure 5.01 Example of an extended interpersonal skill – cues and clues

The following exchange taken from the transcript of Dr C consulting with Margaret Henderson provides an illustration of personalised expertise:

Doctor: *Have you had any other investigations done on your back?*

Patient: *No. No.*

Doctor: *What do you feel has been the root cause of it? Have you any experience of back trouble? Have you any ideas yourself of where it has come from or . . .?*

The doctor here uses an open question, a closed question and another open question followed by the invitational 'or' – as a combined question – to illustrate the desired answer. This type of questioning forms one aspect of this doctor's consulting style.

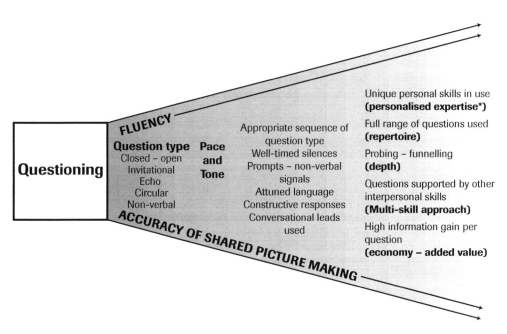

Figure 5.02 Example of an extended interpersonal skill – questioning

The attempt in Figure 5.01 to show how a specific skill might progress, however exploratory, should make it apparent that skills can be used in more sophisticated ways to respond to the needs of patients. It is even possible that the language used to describe what might happen, as in Figures 5.01 and 5.02, may also suggest how expertise development might be attempted.

For example Hargie and Dickson consider in depth non-verbal communication, questioning, listening, explaining and negotiating skills.[5] They consider how skilled behaviours are developed from groupings of multiple skills. It should be clear from Figure 5.02 how skilled behaviours directed to clinical tasks are related to basic interpersonal skills. In addition, the more developed the grouping of skills, the more effective the skilled behaviours.

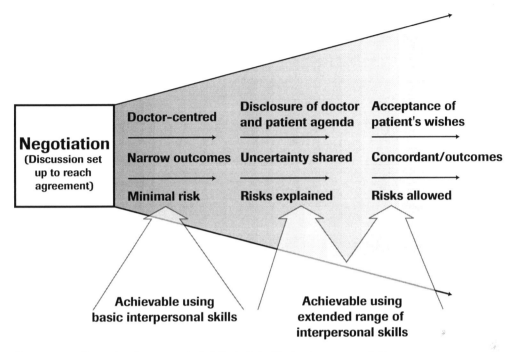

Figure 5.03 Example of an extended skilled clinical behaviour – negotiation

It should be emphasised that diagrams of this kind are drawn to encourage dialogue – they are learning diagrams. They are not intended to portray any conclusive conception of, in this case, negotiation. Their purpose at one level is to draw attention to the multidimensional dynamic of any skill or skilled behaviour and at another to encourage similar consideration to be applied to expertise development.

The extent to which in-depth consideration of skilled behaviour and associated skills can impact on consultation quality is well illustrated by the work of Tim Norfolk, which focuses on the role of empathy and other communication skills in establishing and maintaining therapeutic rapport.[6] In a similar way, Simon Cocksedge has explored ways in which listening can be extended as a distinct therapeutic approach in primary care surgeries, particularly with anxious and depressed patients.[7]

The interpersonal skills overview illustrates the link between the interpersonal skills segment of the consulting skills circle at the centre of the Consultation Expertise Model and higher levels of consulting expertise. We believe this aspect of expertise along with similar developments in medical knowledge and skill and problem framing and solving will develop in parallel and in support of clinical effectiveness.

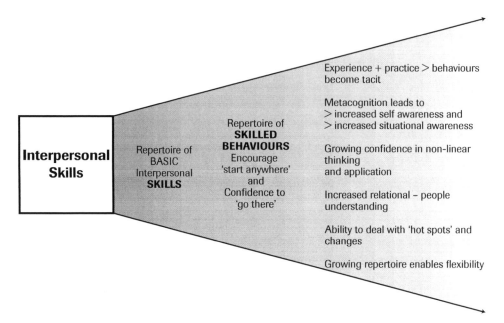

Figure 5.04 Example of an interpersonal skills overview

KEY CONCEPTS IN RELATION TO THE IMPRESSION GRAPH
Understanding intuition

> *'Intuition is a decision-making method that is used unconsciously by experienced practitioners but is inaccessible to the novice. It is rapid, subtle, contextual, and does not follow simple cause-and-effect logic.'*[8]

Why do I feel so tired when dealing with this patient? Why do I want to bury myself in the computer instead of engaging with this patient? Why am I on a mission for this patient? What sort of a game have I got into here?

Recognising the clues is the first step, and understanding what they mean is the next. Pattern recognition often appears both easy and fast in expert consulters – this is because reasoning has become fluent and intuitive. They can bring this awareness to consciousness even while heavily intellectually engaged elsewhere. Imagine we're listening to a complicated story, anxious not to miss that vital piece of history that will make sense of it all. Then up from our unconscious comes a little voice saying 'This is all irrelevant, it isn't the patient's real agenda!' or 'Whoops, we've just skated past the important bit!' Of course, it may not only be the patient's behaviour that gives us the clues, but also our own. A lot of us get these feelings but aren't quick enough to realise them intellectually or to start acting on them. In some instances, we don't have enough confidence or trust in our intuition to use it.

What, though, is intuition? 'Intuition is the ability to receive or assimilate knowledge by direct perception – to know immediately without reasoning' (*New Shorter English Dictionary*).

Moreover, intuition as applied in the family doctor consultation is as dependent upon local-level insights into patient behaviour (interpersonal expertise) as it is on clinical expertise. It is dependent upon years of interaction with many, many patients of all shapes, sizes, personalities and cultural differences, presenting with an extensive range of health problems. Intuition differs from opinion since intuition is a way of experiencing events, while opinion is based on that experience. Intuition also differs from instinct, which does not necessarily have the experiential element at all. A person who has an intuitive basis for an opinion probably cannot immediately fully explain why he or she holds that view; however, a person may later rationalise an intuition by developing a chain of logic to demonstrate more structurally why the intuition is valid.

Intuition gives us the ability to trust in our own unconscious processes and respond to gut feeling. However, reflection, restructuring and reformulating need to occur alongside our intuition as hypotheses are tested out. The latter needs to occur because judgement errors occur as a natural consequence of limitations in our cognitive capacities and because of the human tendency to adopt heuristics (shortcuts) in reasoning. To quote Nyiri:

> *Human experts gradually absorb a repertory of working rules of thumb, or heuristics, that combined with book knowledge, make them expert practitioners.*[9]

Regular reflective thinking is essential to gain confidence and awareness to enable us to apply intuitive pattern recognition at expert level.

But how is it possible to intuitively gather the necessary information in such a short time? Intuition and pattern recognition are intimately linked. To be a successful decision-maker, we have to edit. The answer is that our unconscious engages in 'thin slicing', which is a critical component of rapid cognition. 'Thin slicing'[10] refers to the ability of our unconscious to find patterns in situations and behaviour based on very narrow slices of experience. Our internal computer effortlessly and instantly finds a pattern in chaos. If we could not thin slice and make sense of complicated situations in a flash, complex processes, for example, would be chaotic.

Primary care practitioners also combine information from a wide range of sources into 'mindlines' (internalised, collectively reinforced tacit guidelines) which they use to inform their practice.[11] Mindlines are more complex than the heuristics and 'rules of thumb', as they are not simple short-cuts. They are learned, internalised sequences of thought and behaviour that again, practitioners find difficult to articulate.

The Impression Graph dimension draws a line from mechanistic to intuitive to reflect the initial training needed to use routines and protocols to ensure that appropriate medical decisions are made. In this sense 'clinical method'[12] is a mechanistic approach. It is also worth considering whether the 'hypothetico-deductive' approach isn't an important precedent for the development of intuitive consulting. It should be understood that family doctors switch from intuitive reactions to deliberation very quickly when evidence conflicts with tacit thinking. Seamlessly, they may return to more rational, more mechanistic, evidence-seeking approaches. Family doctors talk about reverting to thinking more deliberately when they feel uneasy, when they don't know what's going on and when they're out of the comfort zone or faced with something entirely new. Intuition is a way of knowing what has particular value when dealing with complex patient cases. Intuitive thinking can be spotted when a consultation seems easy and not dominated by heavy clinical questioning; knights'-move thinking misses out on detail and the whole picture of consulting may appear fluent. Doctors who rely on a degree of intuition can freewheel and accept information more randomly, knowing that they can make and check out judgements.

Patients' lifeworld

Imagine for a moment running a videotape of your last consultation backwards: the patient leaves the consulting room, closes the door with a knock and disappears into the corridor. How much do we know about what people think about as they come towards the surgery door? As they disappear through the front door of the surgery, what kind of a world are they returning to? As they back into their cars in the car park, how are they readjusting themselves to present their problems to the receptionist so as to get an appointment today? What kind of family environment have they left behind: what does their spouse think about seeking help for a problem which mother-in-law could have sorted in no time? How will their employer react to being told that they will arrive later for work and that further time off may be necessary?

As family doctors, we are used to meeting people in an environment over which we have control. We have been involved probably in the design of the physical space. We have moved the computer to a place that suits us. We have chosen the size and height of our chair and control where the patient can sit down. We control how much time people can spend with us. Sometimes we carefully control the way that people talk to us in the consultation so that we obtain a 'good history' that we can share with other doctors.

We have to behave in this way in order to be able to function professionally. We are trained, carefully and expensively, to work efficiently and effectively. As a consequence, we have developed all sorts of procedures and practices that we hardly notice any more – we take them for granted as normal behaviour. We have created our own professional world of structures, procedures, behaviour and language. It is our **medical world,** a world of professionally shared meanings and values. It is not a world which is so meaningful to our patients as they journey from their world of work relationships and different sets of family values.

Each patient that comes to see us brings a highly individual and personalised world view. Parts may be shared with family, colleagues or other social groups, but equally they may not be. It is an individual **patient lifeworld.**

The concept of lifeworld arises from the branch of philosophy known as phenomenology. If you are curious about this, try entering 'Lifeworld' into a Google search. Lifeworld was introduced into healthcare largely through the work of EG Mischler, who emphasised the importance of meanings in particular contexts.[13] This can work both ways: context can impose meaning – for example the requirement to enter disease codes into a computer register can limit the ways we understand what a patient tells us about their problem in real life. In addition, there may be multiple meanings possible in a particular context: to a child their father's toolbox can be a wonderful source of imaginative play. Child and father will place different meanings on the importance of mixing screws or blunting chisels.

Narrative medicine talks about **history building** to describe the process of developing shared understanding in the consultation between the medical world and patient lifeworld.[14] History building requires sensitive attention to the narrative and the sharing of tentative understandings before negotiating a way forward and agreeing an outcome.

Here is one patient story. You might like to think how you could respond to this story to help in the care of this patient.

> *'The worst part of having seizures is knowing that they can happen anytime and even though drugs control mine most of the time they occasionally break through. Just realising that can happen has been a difficult fact to accept as for many years I tried to hide it from anyone else, thinking they would judge me in a way that would cross me off their list as a friend for sure. Gradually I have learned that people aren't like that and I don't have to fear their judgement and it has opened a lot of doors which I had previously closed on myself. I am now a massage therapist and have no fear in telling my clients that I do get seizures occasionally and what they should do if this happens.'*[15]

You may wish to explore the website 'healthtalkonline'[16] for stories that patients tell about tensions between the medical world and patient lifeworld.

> *'Mischler (1984) described two contrasting voices; the voice of medicine and the voice of the lifeworld. The voice of medicine on the one hand, promotes a*

scientific detached attitude and uses questions such as; "Where does it hurt?",
"When did it start?", "How long does it last?", "What makes it better or worse?".
The voice of the lifeworld, on the other hand, reflects a "common sense" view of
the world. It centres on the individual's particular social context, the meaning
of illness events and how these may affect the achievement of personal goals.
Typical questions to ask in exploring the lifeworld are: "What are you most
concerned about?", "How does it disrupt your life?", "What do you think it
is?", "How do you think I can help you?" [17]

You can tell whether the patient lifeworld has been adequately incorporated into the
shared understanding by looking at the following areas of the Model:

- Impression Graph (columns 2–3): how much of the wider context is
  discussed and used in developing shared understanding?
- Respecting Patients: how much is understood about the patient's ideas,
  concerns and expectations?
- Focus: how are the cues and clues responded to?

KEY CONCEPTS IN RELATION TO EXPERTISE TRAINING
Starting anywhere

We have already presented the development of expertise as a process that builds
upon existing skills to develop craft mastery. The process is driven by curiosity, perceptiveness and attention to detail, and it requires commitment to reflective change.
How this process works may be seen from the following story.

After 15 years as a family doctor and more than 10 as a teacher of 'communication skills'
to students and family doctor registrars, one of us changed the way he opened the
consultation with patients in the surgery. This unanticipated change of behaviour followed
a workshop facilitated by a dietician aimed at changing the way clinicians spoke with obese
patients. After a role play with another participant, the feedback had been positive until
the role player commented that the consultation was lost as soon as the doctor had asked,
'What can I do to help you today?' The answer was, 'I don't know and I can't tell you and
it probably isn't in your power anyway!' Not something that patients feel able to say very
often and, in this case, the 'patient' didn't either. So they talked about something else while
the role player undermined all the doctor's 'helpful' suggestions – with some glee it turned
out later in feedback.

In the doctor's head this feedback chimed with something he had read about the
way smokers respond to attempts to modify their smoking habits. Maybe it applied
to wider groups of people. How else could he put it? What was it about the words he

had used that sank the rapport? Surely a couple of words couldn't be that important? During the rest of the workshop he tried some new formulations and finally when he couldn't think of anything new to try, said nothing.

Back in the surgery, the differences were startling. He heard new things from patients he thought he knew well over many years. Frequently it became necessary to revise his view of their personality or help-seeking behaviour. Patients became even more interesting. But what was going on?

He tried to present his conclusions at an appraisal to an appraiser who didn't seem to be a reflective type but made many suggestions – nearly all now forgotten. He remembers thinking 'This appraiser is quite skilful really but he doesn't really care about how this affects me personally as a professional.'

That was the key. Expression of the personal is important, whether in appraisal or other consultations. But we all knew that. For years this doctor had been 'helping' students learn how to address the patient lifeworld, and for years they had been telling him that it was for them a risky business; too time-consuming and inefficient with no apparent rewards in management outcomes. As one trainee put it after a workshop on patient-centred skills: 'This is all very interesting but when I get into practice I will have to use the old efficient questioning or I shall never keep to time.' That's almost certainly true. A relevant skill has been learned but not yet the experience to make it count.

The problem is that changing the words that help us maintain control and direction of the consultation allows the patient to move into our professionally uncertain or unfamiliar areas. We have referred to the willingness to follow as 'going there'.[18] Unless we are prepared to follow, the significance of the story may be missed. If we miss the significance, then we will struggle with 'concordance' and hence outcomes.

One of the differences that struck our colleague was in the way that people told their stories. Sometimes it was unclear why they had come to see him as a doctor. The story might start with a report of another conversation or a discussion about the weather. People would start anywhere they felt like and meander about until they decided what the problems were. Terribly inefficient – maybe the trainee was right.

But maybe efficiency is an inappropriate quality by which to judge story-telling. We keep going on about that how interpersonal behaviour in the consultation is complex as well as complicated on occasions. Efficiency can be applied to the complicated elements of a consultation but not to the complex. Medical case histories are an established and efficient way of communicating the technically complicated process of medical thinking. We need the structure to understand the clinical thought processes.

The lifeworld stories patients tell in the consultation are complex. Meaning emerges from them on occasions only slowly. In these situations the starting point sometimes cannot be defined, yet start we must. What our colleague discovered was that when combined with his experience, the starting point was not critical. Stories could be told backwards, forwards with loops or flashbacks and often not in a linear time sequence. It was, however, critical to listen for gaps and to ensure that the story had an ending – at least for the time being. For an experienced consulter it is safe to start anywhere, i.e. wherever the patient wants.

Training for 'starting anywhere'
It should be clear from the following pages that 'starting anywhere', 'going there' and 'concordance' are overlapping concepts. Each will embody elements of the others, and any programme of expertise development will need to address all three.

'Starting anywhere', remember, does not require new skills but the refashioning of the use to which skills are put in the light of experience so far. It might mean allowing learners to take risks. Role plays and simulations may make this less stressful for the participants.

Some doctors prefer to evolve their behaviour in partnership with their patients. One doctor we know tells of how one day, when completely stuck in a consultation, he asked if the patient were willing to try something that the doctor had never done before. They then swapped places and functions, the doctor struggling to find understanding from the patient's perspective while the patient explored ways forward from the doctor's chair. A rather dramatic approach, but you could not accuse this doctor of shirking the responsibility to 'transform holistic understanding into practical measures', to quote the RCGP Curriculum for General Practice again.

Going there

The phrase 'going there' was seized upon as a means of pinpointing a highly significant point in the consultation, a point that, while it may be implicit in a range of consultation models, in our experience is not part of training language.[19] It refers to a critical point at which the consultation goes far deeper into the nature of the patient's story *with a view to treatment and management*. A point at which a family doctor trainee particularly and other doctors may possibly go beyond their comfort zone into a realm of uncertainty outside biomedical parameters. The ability to 'go there' and deal with whatever issues arise in a constructive therapeutic manner equates with expert behaviour. For example:

The patient wanted a repeat prescription for fluoxetine.

Doctor: (Good I could do with a quick consultation; don't like getting behind.) *Well, how are you?*

Patient: *I'm getting better thank you.*

Doctor: *You've now been on two months, so how much better are you?*

> Works with the individuality of the patient.
> **Respecting patients**

Patient: *Oh, about 70 percent.*

Doctor: *Good, you're getting there then.* (There is something wrong, the smile is not right, it's a bit false and she's not meeting my gaze; well she is depressed so perhaps not surprising, so just press the key for the fluoxetine, but, oh no, I'm opening my big mouth). *How are you coping then?* (I know her quite well, early 30s with two young children and relationship broke up a while ago, which surprised me as she seemed cheerful and bubbly).

> Uses emotional affect of patient as diagnostic tool.
> **Synthesising skills**

Patient: *All right.* (Doesn't sound it).

Doctor: *So what got you down?*

Patient: *I don't know, I just started feeling down, felt alone.*

Doctor: (Alone, thought she had a close family who would give support). *Have you talked with your family about how you feel?*

Patient: *No, I haven't talked with anyone.*

Doctor: *That sounds difficult, keeping it all to yourself, locked out.* (She's reacted to 'locked out', very uneasy, looking down and away. Silence . . . uh, I've met this before). *You don't have to answer this, but have you ever been abused, sexually?*

> Ability to recognise patterns in most situations/confidence in own judgement.
> **Recognising patterns**

The reaction is profound, with head in hands, and there is silence for the next 10 minutes. It ends with her able to look at me and smile, a proper one. Nothing is acknowledged but she agrees she would like to be referred to a counsellor.

But what about when you have not been such an able doctor, and you're feeling a little less then proud of yourself?

They had been a close couple, and I should have admitted her earlier with the chest pain despite her protestations that she didn't want to go in. We have the power to persuade people as to what is in their best interests and sometimes we should use it. I didn't, she deteriorated, was admitted later and died. I wasn't looking forward to seeing him with guilt lurking around and, yes, he was angry in his grief. The consultation could have gone on in a stiff formal way but I went there, the anger was acknowledged, the guilt exposed. He did well with counselling and still sees me.

Perhaps the most difficult part is to be aware of the problems within that impede us in going there. The problems may include fear of provoking anger; fear of not being able to contain the emotion; desire to avoid conflict; and not wanting to embarrass, dominate or protect. These will have their origins in our past. And how are we going to be aware of those influences? Perhaps by being aware of the inner voice, being prepared to acknowledge mistakes or deficiencies when things don't go right and honestly reflect on them, getting ourselves educated, and perhaps above all, sharing these issues with others.

Concordance

The achievement of concordance (when appropriate) requires clinical acumen and highly developed interpersonal behaviours. It is not easy. Because its achievement in all its patient manifestations equates with expert consulting behaviour, a concordance repertoire is considered to be vital for expertise growth.

The concept of concordance was explored in the report *From Compliance to Concordance*.[20] It was principally concerned with the well-documented concern of high non-compliance with prescribed medications. In an attempt to understand why patients behaved in this way, it changed the focus from the doctor, their professional expertise and giving of medical advice to the patient and their knowledge, concerns and experience of illness (*see* Going there, p.156). It suggested in normal circumstances, the patients' preferences regarding treatment should be given priority over those of the doctor. In practice it is the patient who makes the final decision whether to take the medication. This decision may be made on very different criteria from those of the medical profession. Consequently, this sharing of experience, exchange of ideas, learning from one another and relationship between the family practitioner and patient throughout the consultation is paramount in concordance.[21]

> Balances patient and doctor need as appropriate.
> **Synthesising skills**

'From the professional perspective non-compliant patient behaviour appears irrational and intransigent and poses an enduring puzzle.'[22]

The concept of concordance may challenge our expectation and skills in consulting as a family practitioner, and there may be difficulties in its implementation. It is not synonymous with compliance, patient education or being well informed. Patient education will not necessarily mean the patient will make the correct decision, at least in the doctor's eyes. Decisions may be at odds with cost-effectiveness and have quality target issues. Giving information is usually beneficial in informing patients but can be a problem in confusing and conflicting with their expectations. Knowledge implies responsibility, and patients do not always want to assume an active role, which is particularly likely in serious or terminal illness. Living life may be more important than learning the necessarily difficult information to make painful decisions, and so their delegation is therefore returned to the doctor.

Risk is notoriously difficult to calculate, and even where measured accurately means different things to different people, in different contexts and in its presentation. A reduction of risk of 50% may encourage acceptance of treatments, but not if it means a reduction of 1 in 10 000 to 1 in 20 000. Also choice of several treatments, sometimes of marginal or uncertain outcome benefits, may exist. It is not uncommon for the patient to delegate the decision to the doctor: 'You're the doctor, you decide.'

> Explains what evidence suggests and where risks lie.
> **Dealing with uncertainty**

Evidence-based medicine attempts to remove idiosyncratic clinical decisions but may conflict with patient-centred medicine. Awareness of the patient's experience of illness and appreciation of patient values in juxtaposition with doctor preferences is paramount in such cases.

'Limiting the application of concordance to medicines merely marginalises its relevance, rather than conferring a distinctive identity. The choice might refer to no treatment, or drugs as one among several possible options. It is consultations and relationships that are concordant, not just discussion or decisions about medicines.'[23]

An example is the poor compliance in elderly people to the long-term taking of statins. Their taking may be evidence-based but may imply illness or dependency whilst otherwise well.

> 'The key issue for patients is centred on illness acceptance rather than medicines use.'[24]

Doctors are also bad at altering their own behaviour, even in response to logic. Hand washing can reduce the spread of healthcare-associated infection, but they still do not wash their hands.

Concordance increases the challenge for both doctor and patient, opening up the possibility of disagreement and conflict. This may explain the reluctance of both parties to accept it. While patients want to be 'fully informed', what this constitutes remains uncertain. Nor are patients' preferences uniform. The wish to know every detail of risks and complications of surgery or side effects of drugs testify to this. The way in which individuals process expert knowledge is uncertain; some is immediately forgotten and some incorrectly retained. These are challenges indeed, not only for the competent to proficient consulter but also for the expert.

> Involves patient in understanding management options in all problem areas.
> **Focus**

Patients still value the consultation, despite the internet and other sources of information. The competent or proficient doctor will listen and explain. The expert doctor will know information does not substitute for empathy. Listening and encouraging the patient to discuss their experience of illness, personal and other, are paramount to how they wish to proceed. This will entail sensitivity to each patient as an individual and having the skills to sense the differing levels of participation and wish for control over the proceedings. This will be aided over time as the doctor continues to share unfolding life stories.

> Shares and uses own **and** patient's ideas, concerns and expectations.
> **Respecting patients**

> 'The real goal of concordant consultation is that all parties exchange information, and share different perspectives as the basis of an increased

understanding. This is primarily focussed on the relationship between patients and professional rather than a specific outcome of the consultation.'[25]

The concordance divide

Using the principles of concordance as performance criteria allows family doctors to be distinguished as:

- doctors who do not espouse concordant outcomes
- doctors who espouse concordance but subvert the principle by aiming for 'informed compliance' (i.e. sharing more information but avoiding patients' ideas and feelings and thus avoiding the problems associated with truthful agreements) – and thus limit themselves to levels of proficiency
- doctors who espouse concordant outcomes and as a consequence confront the many difficult issues, both medical and personal, that this involves – but thereby open up the potential for expert behaviour.

In summary

Concordance has been selected as an expertise concept because:

1. concordant consultation outcomes are by definition patient-centred in a manner consistent with the expert performance level in the Consultation Expertise Model and the upper reaches of the Impression Graph
2. concordance as a desired consultation outcome allows consideration of complex issues which require in-depth understanding
3. concordance demands a high level of interpersonal skill, a secure knowledge base and flexible problem-solving. Informing the patient of risks and opportunities is just one aspect, and this requires meaningful communication of clinical significance, personal significance and, of course, significance regarding practice targets.

References

1. Elwyn G, Gwyn R. Stories we hear and stories we tell: analysing talk in clinical practice. *BMJ*. 1999; **318**: 188.
2. Elwyn G. *Shared Decision Making: patient involvement in clinical practice*. Nijmegan: WOK; 2001.
3. Hargie O, editor. *Handbook of Communication Skills*. 3rd ed. London: Routledge; 2006. p. 8.
4. Maguire P. *Communication Skills For Doctors*. London: Arnold; 2000. p. 5.
5. Hargie O, Dickson D. *Skilled Interpersonal Communication: research, theory and practice*. 4th ed. London: Routledge; 2006.
6. Norfolk T, Birdi K, Walsh D. The role of empathy in establishing rapport in the consultation: a new model. *Med Educ*. 2007; **41**: 690–7.

7. Cocksedge S. *Listening as Work in Primary Care.* Oxford: Radcliffe Medical Press; 2005.

8. Greenhalgh T. Intuition and evidence – uneasy bedfellows? *Br J Gen Pract.* 2002; **52**: 396–400.

9. Nyiri J. Traditional and practical knowledge. In: Nyiri J, Barry S, editors. *Outlines of a Theory of Traditions and Skills.* London: Croom; 1988.

10. Gladwell M. *Blink: the power of thinking without thinking.* London: Allen Lane – Penguin Books; 2005.

11. Gabbay J, Lemay A. Evidence based guidelines or collectively constructed 'Mindlines'? Ethnographic study of knowledge management in primary care. *BMJ.* 2004; **329**; 1013.

12. Fraser R. *Clinical Method: a general practice approach.* Oxford: Butterworth-Heinmann; 1987.

13. Mischler E. *Discourse of Medicine: dialectics on medical interviews.* Norwood, NJ: Ablex; 1984.

14. Barry C, Stevenson F, Britten N, *et al.* Giving voice to the lifeworld. More humane, more effective medical care? A qualitative study of doctor-patient communication in general practice. *Soc Sci Med.* 2001; **53**: 487–505.

15. Schachter SC. Quoted in Houston, M. *The Role of Narrative in Healthcare.* Commissioned by the Arts Council for the Arts and Health Conference, Dublin Castle; 2004. Available at: www.artscouncil.ie/Publications/ahc_MuirisHouston_essay.rtf (accessed 12 August 2008).

16. www.healthtalkonline.org (accessed 24 October 2008).

17. Brown JB, Stewart M, Weston WW. *Challenges and Solutions in Patient Centred Care: a case book.* Oxford: Radcliffe Medical Press; 2002. p. 1.

18. Ashton L, Worrall P. Going there. *Educ Prim Care.* 2008; **19**: 84–9.

19. Ibid.

20. Marinker M. From Compliance to Concordance: a personal view. In: Bond C, editor. *Concordance: a partnership in medicine-taking.* London: Pharmaceutical Press; 2004.

21. Ibid.

22. Pollack K. *Concordance in Medical Consultations.* Oxford: Radcliffe Medical Press; 2005. p. 9.

23. Ibid. p. 67.

24. Ibid. p. 59.

25. Ibid. p. 149.

6 PRACTICAL APPROACHES TO DEVELOPING ADVANCED CONSULTING EXPERTISE

ESTABLISHING A MINDSET AND DIRECTION OF TRAVEL

Given a desire to keep life as clear and uncluttered as possible, we suggest that progression to higher levels of consulting expertise can be facilitated in two ways:

1. achieving a **mindset** that enables maximum benefit to be gained from day-to-day experience
2. being clear about the **direction of travel** and what to pay attention to in the field of expertise development while using the Consultation Expertise Model as a staging-post framework.

Mindset

> *'"Mental models" are deeply ingrained assumptions, generalisations, or even pictures or images that influence how we understand the world and how we take action.'*[1]

Having an expertise focus

It was emphasised earlier that advanced consulting is about the development of existing skills. That remains the case. Indeed, **expertise is best thought of in 'craft terms'** of building on previous skill, of attending to the brush strokes of clinical application, of variation in the pace and tone of the patient episode and of creative phrasing, i.e. the detail that only comes from practice. Consulting expertise development lies in the detail of nuance, of timing, of situational awareness (*see* p. 54), of word choice and in similar attributes that can be explored with nothing more taxing than curiosity. Difficult though it may be to swallow, it is these details that can make the difference between good and bad outcomes. Think of the very knowledgeable, skilled clinician who, because he or she looks uninterested, fails to elicit a critical disclosure. In the words of John Dewey, it is 'the attention to detail that ensures mastery over the means of execution.'[2] In the terminology of the RCGP Curriculum for General Practice, expertise development should be focused on a sophisticated extension of what, in Domain 6, are listed as, 'The skills to transform holistic understanding into practical measures'.[3] **Expertise lies in the detail of 'complex human systems'.**

> 'The problem-solving mindset can be adequate for technical problems. But it can be woefully inadequate for complex human systems, where problems often arise from the unquestioned assumptions of deeply habitual ways of acting.'[4]

Having a commitment

There is no escaping the individual nature of family doctor consulting. Add to that the fact that, so far, there is little pressure or encouragement to engage voluntarily on a quest for high levels of expertise (proficient is adequate enough?). So why bother? The answer to that must lie in whatever intrinsic reward individual practitioners value – increased self-esteem? – personal mastery? – job satisfaction? – teaching ambition? – better outcomes for patients?

Taking control of the experience

> 'It is in this interplay between expectation and experience that learning occurs. In Hegel's phrase, "Any experience that does not violate expectation is not worthy of the name of experience."'[5]

If violating expectations sounds overly dramatic, it is self-evident that concentrating on the detail of practice (for example, concentrating on how you pick up, acknowledge and prioritise cues and clues) may extend over months, if not years. The pace of experiential learning is likely to vary considerably. There will be times when private or professional life pressures take over. Even so, there may be some learning if there is a long-term learning plan. Learning may result from a passing thought – 'I didn't check whether he understood' – checking is still relevant at expert level but maybe in a different manner and style – you may subsequently find you are checking more deliberately. It's useful to remember, 'all learning is re-learning' (Kolb again). Expertise development is for the long haul. By definition, the transition to intuitive practice takes time.

Learning from experience requires deliberate attention

> 'Practice alone does not make perfect. It is practice, the results of which are known, understood and acted upon, that improves skill.'[6]

Experience cannot be fast-tracked

> 'There is a well established "10-year rule" in relation to learning complex skill routines, in that the highest level of performance in any field is only attained after 10 years of concerted practice and training.'[7]

Response to experience

> 'There are two main impediments to gaining experience: standing on one's dignity, which fogs the mind with smoke, and timidity, which in the face of danger discourages.'[8]

Benefiting from experience depends upon interplay between the following factors: knowing how your learning style fits with everyday practice and your lifestyle. You will probably know how you learn best and how best you can squeeze in some personal learning. The problem is actually doing it and finding time to reflect on it.

Organising learning support

As we know only too well, family doctor consulting, despite all the human inter-action in the surgery, is a solitary professional activity. A serious downside of this is a powerful reticence, for some, to expose consultations to more open scrutiny. Unfortunately, for most of us there are limits to self-coaching; we need feedback from colleagues. Though it is possible to record and fingerprint consultations solo, it is far more beneficial to exchange and receive feedback from colleagues. Identifying blind spots alone is difficult and overcoming them without help even more difficult. Looking at tapes and fingerprinting with colleagues is ideal because the to and fro of discussion may not only lead to more insightful feedback and longer-term learn-ing, it can also be more companionable. Admittedly, arranging support is not always easy, particularly in practices where there is reticence about exposing what goes on in the consulting room.

> 'The educational research literature suggests that we can improve our intui-tive powers through systematic critical reflection about intuitive judgements – for example, through creative writing and dialogue with professional colleagues.'[9]

The working situation may help or hinder the development of expertise. Peter Senge, who we have already quoted, is best known for promoting the idea of the 'learning organisation'. Such organisations actively encourage 'open' discussion of practice, whole-team discussion of practice protocols, time out to learn and other means whereby everybody both grows in expertise and collaborates in providing a better quality of healthcare.

> *'Personal mastery is the discipline of continually clarifying and deepening our personal vision, of focussing our energies, of developing patience, and of seeing reality objectively. As such, it is an essential cornerstone of the learning organisation – the learning organisation's spiritual foundation. An organisation's commitment to and capacity for learning, can be no greater than that of its members.'*[10]

It is the 'closed' practices, where there is limited discussion and little tolerance of risk and where disclosure of weakness or fault is constrained, that minimise the potential for expertise growth. In some practices the partners may be so busy that 'laissez faire' applies; do as you wish. To some extent, therefore, the nature of the working environment will determine individual learning plans and, for instance, whether colleague support is arranged internally or externally.

Incorporate the environmental opportunities and constraints into the learning plan
A focus on the consultation should not preclude other learning opportunities such as courses, e-learning, training as a practitioner with a special interest (PwSI), part-time work in secondary care specialisms or community placements, all of which may have an expertise spin-off.

Be prepared to refocus

> *'The notion that expertise is associated with a qualitative transition from a conceptually rich and rational knowledge base to one comprised of largely experiential and non-analytical instances is a radical departure from conventional views of clinical competence.'*[11]

There will be times when a major shift of behaviour might be indicated.

> *'. . . as clinical careers develop [doctors] change their intellectual orientation, integrate and sort out knowledge and refocus their decision making on a different basis than the process oriented one they were taught.'*[12]

We have already mentioned the 'qualitative leap' required to accommodate a patient-centred approach: a leap from a linear, more predictable type of thinking within a biomedical envelope to one that is a non-linear, less predictable type of thinking that will address the biomedical and biographical elements of the consultation in tandem. The expertise journey may present more such leaps; recognising that one is working more intuitively may be one.

> *'There is a difference between a deepening of the mind – as occurs when one learns more about a subject or enhances one's skills – and a genuine*

transformation of mind, when one's knowledge or skill veer in a new direction.'[13]

Taking reflection seriously

Quality of reflection = quality of learning = behaviour change = expertise.

> *'... personal mastery, is not something you possess, it is a process. It is a lifelong discipline. People with high levels of personal mastery are acutely aware of their ignorance, their incompetence, their growth areas. And they are deeply self-confident. Paradoxical? Only for those who do not see that "the journey is the reward".'*[14]

Think of expertise development as a journey.

Direction of travel

Focus of travel

Simply stated, the direction of travel is onwards to that moment in time when consulting becomes routinely easy: easy to the point when it is possible to sit down with most patients, as skilled musicians do with a score, and perform uniquely and memorably (for audience or patient) without apparent effort.

It is also a time when new or difficult situations can be faced with a wide repertoire of possible responses. If the end of the journey is as elusive as it sounds, the territory to be travelled is anything but. It is grounded in the detail of everyday experience. That is where the focus needs to be.

A practical travelling framework

> *'Some hopes and ambitions were manifest only as a direction, not a destination. Maybe the trick was to realise you were involved in a process, not aiming at a completely achievable end result, and accept that, but travel hopefully anyway.'*[15]

Starting points

1. Be aware: become comfortable with the idea that advanced family doctor consulting occupies a complex and potentially unpredictable world, built upon but outside the shelter of enclosed biomedically constrained thinking.
2. Be convinced: believe that clinical skills and patient lifeworld skills are of parallel importance for development of expertise.

Guidance

The Consultation Expertise Model provides three kinds of guidance.

1.   Clinical achievement is enabled by development of expertise in the application of medical knowledge and skills, by an increasing facility to frame and solve clinical problems and through sophisticated use of interpersonal skills; encapsulated in the Model as 'consulting skills'.

2.   The indicative statements at expert level, taken collectively, provide a detailed albeit disconnected picture of the behaviours necessary to operate at expert level. These behaviours only become connected in relation to particular cases. Additionally, statements in each of the domains not only offer comparisons related to the level of expertise used in any one consultation, they also present an opportunity to consider what might have been done differently or additionally – a form of feedback. They provide staging (reference) posts. Notwithstanding the inherent difficulty of defining a route to expert level, always mindful that every expert will travel in a uniquely different way, they can provide tangible reference points in the territory to be covered, however that is attempted.

3.   By comparison, the higher-level, more analytical dimensions of the Impression Graph provide a strong lead to the means by which higher-level expertise can be achieved.

Considered together, these three components of the Model provide a guidance framework.

Visiting points

We have limited the expertise journey to development around three all-encompassing learning concepts associated with the Model; these are: 'starting anywhere', 'going there' and achieving (genuinely) concordant outcomes. In-depth exploration of these three concepts has the potential for reflection upon and practice of most of the attributes of the expert practitioner. They can be visited recurrently on a daily basis. In case this sounds insultingly simple, we believe this approach can be justified on three powerful grounds:

1.   the Model assumes a thorough grounding in medicine and consulting practice prior to certification

2.   learning from everyday experience is more likely to be helped by **attention to clear uncluttered concepts** than hindered by more complicated constructs

3.   expertise, as was said at the beginning, does not accrue from new methodology, it grows upon deeper exploration of existing practice.

Tracking development

Performance levels can be tracked routinely:

- by recording and fingerprinting of consultations, on a quarterly or half-yearly basis, for example
- by quick reference to the Impression Graph. This can be done very rapidly immediately after an interesting consultation – 'how would that score?' could be done on an Impression Graph sheet in less than a minute by visiting the concepts
  - 'starting anywhere' – if there is a high level of **intuitive** interaction in the consultation (column 1), reinforced by prompts and probes that require watchful listening, the consultation is bound to start and continue in an unpredictable and maybe jointly controlled fashion, particularly if the consultation starts from an unpredictable point
  - 'going there' – if aspects of the patient's lifeworld play a significant part in the outcomes, particularly longer-term, strategic considerations (columns 2 and 3), this will signify that advanced expertise is in play
  - concordance – the third concept, with its provenance in the well-documented problems of compliance, is inextricably linked to the act of mutually **negotiated** (column 4) management plans. Did the patient leave with an explicitly negotiated management agreement?

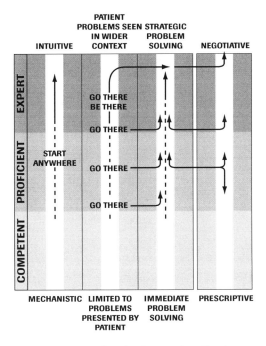

Figure 6.01 Relationship of the 'concepts' to the Impression Graph

Summary: developed expertise and artistry

> *'While there is a large and profoundly important scientific element in the practice of medicine, there is also an indefinable artistry, an imaginative insight, and medicine (they will tell us) is a born marriage between the two.'*[16]

You may have noticed that we haven't talked about artistry so far. That is not because we don't believe that family doctors can demonstrate it, but because we find that it is not a concept that trainees can use to transform their practice. Trainees can recognise much of what they see from experienced practitioners as beyond their existing capabilities, but equally they miss much because it looks too easy or simple.

Instead, we have tried to take the mystery out of the mastery by identifying craft skills relating to domains identified from the practice of experienced clinicians. Craft skills develop out of core skills, and 'mastery' can be enhanced by developing the way that existing skills are integrated and internalised with experience. We have named some important clusters of those integrated skills 'going there', 'starting anywhere' and 'concordance'. These clusters correspond to the axes of the Impression Graph. Expertise has been related to the integration of the clusters in an observably seamless way.

If you are a trainee motivated to mastering your craft, we hope that the Model excites and supports your aspirations. When as a more experienced doctor you can demonstrate wide and consistent expertise, then we think you have some justification in calling yourself an artist in consulting.

DESIGNING AN EXPERTISE TEACHING PROGRAMME: PRELIMINARY THOUGHTS

Chapters have so far been written on an understanding that the Model can be adopted for:

- personally motivated use
- a private or shared reflective dialogue that will result in a potential behaviour change.

The Consultation Expertise Model provides the means to analyse existing consultations with a view to affirming that which is sound, e.g. by identifying expertise staging posts via the indicative statements. And, through dialogue and reflection prompted by fingerprint and Impression Graph statements, to arrive at a decisive next step in the expertise journey, one that can be included in a PDP. Although no doubt aided by trusted colleagues, this is likely to be dependent upon a self-directed, personally motivated learning approach.

Using the Model to design part of a teaching curriculum opens another dimension, that of supporting others in the development of consulting expertise. Such a move into 'taught' mode would involve:

- a shift from a self-directed to a more externally motivated, organised by others form of learning
- the need for programmes to be externally sponsored (e.g. by a primary care trust (PCT), deanery or local RCGP group) with a consequent need for funding
- the prospect of support, guidance and the facility to practise in a safe environment
- the prospect of exposure to a wider realm of colleague experience and contact.

Realisation of such an externally promoted approach would fit well with the notion of improvement based on '*autonomy, mastery, and connectedness*' associated with a policy of '*shifting the whole* [performance] *curve*' of quality improvement.[17]

Using simulators in a teaching programme

It has been assumed from the beginning that the Consultation Expertise Model is predicated on the development of existing skills, not on the imposition of new ways of working. The Model is concerned with providing insights that will in themselves assist the extension of effective and efficient expertise. A teaching programme must therefore build on existing behaviours. Simulated patients provide one such means to do this.

Working with simulated patients has four significant advantages:

1. learning with simulators, either as the consultant or as an observer, inevitably starts with one's current behaviour. Learning is therefore reality-based
2. it is possible to practise – to try out new behaviours more easily and safely than it is in day-to-day practice
3. immediate and honest feedback is available
4. the choice of patient simulation can be contrived to involve important clinical and psycho-social issues.

It is therefore suggested that a teaching programme should, ideally, be structured around workshops using simulated patients with the additional option of using examples from recordings of actual patients. So far the process of consulting has been to a large extent removed from discussion of clinical detail. By using simulated patients and filmed examples, as with fingerprinting real patient cases, the focus continues to be on the seamless interaction of clinical knowledge and skill, medical problem solving and interpersonal skills – the reality.

The starting point for any teaching framework must be based on a sound grounding in consultation models: procedural models, as with Pendleton[18], Neighbour[19],

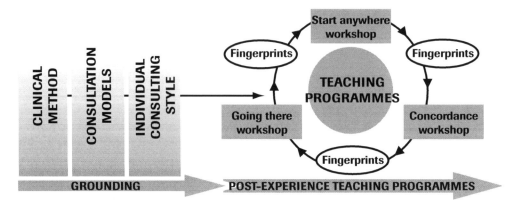

Figure 6.02 Elements in a teaching programme

Cambridge-Calgary[20] or Helman[21], and process-based models, such as the approach developed by Norfolk.[22] These models are used to explore the personal dynamics and increase the structural effectiveness of doctors' individual constructs. Our consulting style emerges from familiarity with publicly recommended consulting models later modified and extended by experience. Fingerprinting procedures then provide not only expertise concepts, but indicators – staging posts for improvement upon which it is possible to integrate the facility to 'start anywhere', to 'go there' and to achieve concordant outcomes.

It is worth repeating that each of these three expertise concepts may be visited daily over many years and that each visit, different for every patient, condition and context, may add valuable know-how.

The three concepts have been chosen because of their profound implications for consulting behaviour change. A teaching workshop based on 'starting anywhere' could, for example, focus literally at a basic level of responding to patients' unpredicted opening statements or at a more profound level of responding intuitively to a patient's demeanour. There is opportunity for a series of workshops at deeper and deeper levels. These workshops are always building and extending previous skills: rapport building and maintenance, identifying and utilising patient's ideas, concerns and expectations and so on. With a clear workshop focus, good case choice and clever facilitation, expertise development for existing practitioners becomes an exciting possibility.

The Model opens up new territory for medical educators.

References

1. Senge P. *The Fifth Discipline*. London: Random House; 1990. p. 6.
2. Dewey J. *Experience and Education*. London: Collier Macmillan; 1938.
3. RCGP. *Curriculum for General Practice: the learning and teaching guide*. London: Royal College of General Practitioners; 2006.
4. Senge P. *Presence: exploring profound change in people, organisations, and society*. London: Nicholas Brealey Publishing; 2005. p. 52.
5. Kolb DA. *Experiential Learning: experience as the source of learning and development*. Englewood Cliffs, NJ: Prentice Hall; 1984. p. 28.
6. Hargie O, editor. *Handbook of Communication Skills*. 3rd ed. London: Routledge; 2006. p. 23.
7. Ibid. p. 12.
8. Erasmus D. *Praise of Folly*. Translated by Clarke R. Richmond: One World Classics; 2008.
9. Greenhalgh T. Intuition and evidence – uneasy bedfellows? *Br J Gen Pract*. 2002; **52**: 396–400.
10. Senge P. *The Fifth Discipline*. London: Random House; 1990. p. 141.
11. Schmidt HG, Norman GR, Boshuizen HPA. A cognitive perspective on medical expertise: theory and implications. *Acad Med*. 1990; **65**(10): 619.
12. Benner P. *From Novice to Expert: excellence and power in clinical nursing practice*. New Jersey: Prentice Hall; 1984.
13. Gardner H. *Changing Minds: the art and science of changing our own and other people's minds*. Boston: Harvard Business School Press; 2006. p. xi.
14. Senge, op cit. p. 6.
15. Banks I. *The Steep Approach to Garbadale*. London: Abacus; 2008. p. 365.
16. Medawar PB. *Induction and Intuition in Scientific Thought*. London: Methuen; 1969. p. 43.
17. Davidoff F. Shame: the elephant in the room. *Qual Saf Health care*. 2002; 11: 2–3.
18. Pendleton D, Schofield T, Tate P, *et al. The New Consultation: developing doctor-patient communication*. Oxford: Oxford University Press; 2003.
19. Neighbour R. *The Inner Consultation*. Newbury: Petroc Press; 1996.
20. Kurtz S, Silverman J, Draper J. *Teaching and Learning Communication Skills in Medicine*. Oxford: Radcliffe Medical Press; 1998.
21. Helman C. *Culture, Health and Illness*. London: Hodder Arnold; 2001.
22. Norfolk T, Birdi K, Walsh D. The role of empathy in establishing rapport in the consultation: a new model. *Med Educ*. 2007; **41**: 690–7.

THE CONSULTATION EXPERTISE MODEL: THE DEVELOPMENTAL JOURNEY

Development of the Model progressed stage by stage over the period 1999 to 2008 as a voluntary process constrained by aspects of participants' lives and changes to family medicine and family doctor training. No initial decision was made to follow an action research process. Only in retrospect did it become apparent that development followed such a process in three clearly defined stages:

1. development phase
2. testing phase
3. dissemination phase.

What follows might best be described as a brief case study.

> 'It should be stressed that action research concerns actual, not abstract pictures. It involves learning about the real, material, concrete, particular practices of particular people in particular places.'[1]

1. Development phase

> **Question:** What are the higher-order skills in the consultation, how might they best be identified and, ultimately, how might we best educate for them?

Action

- **Letter of invitation** – The director of GP postgraduate training circulates a letter asking family doctor trainers to volunteer as members of a group with a remit to explore the nature of higher-order expertise – nine respond.
- **Discussion** – Eight volunteers meet and agree, after several meetings watching videotapes of each other consulting and discussing surrounding issues, on a series of skill **domains** and assumptions relevant to higher-order

consulting. These are incorporated into a linear model (*See* Figure A.1). This Model is based on a projection of clinical method and a sequence of **performance progression** derived from the work of the Dreyfus brothers and illustrated with five different approaches to the same case (*See* Figure A.2).

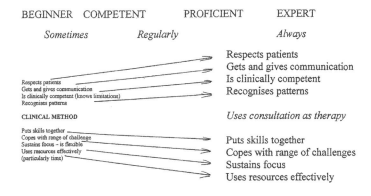

Figure A.1 The linear model

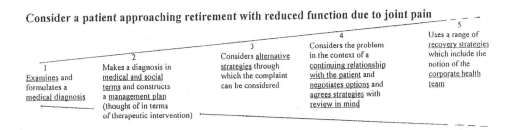

Figure A.2 Illustration of case treatment progression

'It is . . . participatory in the sense that people can only do action research "on" themselves – individually or collectively. It is not research done on others.'[2]

● **Exposure** of work in progress – the linear model is presented to colleagues at the annual Deanery Trainers' Conference. Feedback indicates that:
  — there is resistance to the very idea of identifying higher-order consulting
  — there is a view that the Leicester Assessment Package (LAP) already provides an answer to the question
  — the linear model is too complicated
  — using a circular format to present the ideas in the linear model might be preferable.

INSIGHT – Consultation **fingerprints** can be drawn using the circular model.

Question: Do experienced doctors' consultations differ from those of advanced beginners and newly certificated competent doctors according to case fingerprints?

Action

- **Research** – Research is conducted into how medical students and doctors at different experience levels consult. Two fourth-year medical students, two GP specialty training registrars (GPStR), two new family doctors and two long-experienced family doctors each consult with three simulated patients (SPs).

  The 24 consultations (eight consulters and three patients) are marked using the circular model categories and evidence from the videotaped consultations and patient rating scales (PRS). SPs are trained to use the PRSs for the national simulated patient surgeries for summative assessment.
  - the results reflect differences according to experience, as anticipated
  - there are differences between the performances of each pair – Figure A.3
  - performance by the same doctor varies from patient to patient
  - the PRSs designed to assess minimum competence for certification provide little useful evidence for understanding experienced doctor fingerprints
  - the fingerprints are too dependent on subjective judgement.

INSIGHT – Fingerprints need a more objective means to distinguish between case performances on the competent to expert spectrum. The idea of behavioural frequency is introduced.

Question: How do experienced doctors perform in normal surgery situations with real patients as identified by consultation fingerprints?

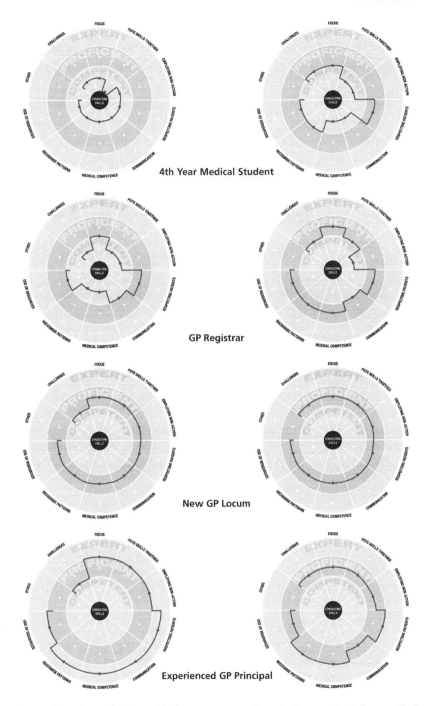

Fingerprints of consultations with the same two medium-challenge patients by a medical student/doctors at different experience levels

Figure A.3 Fingerprints showing variation at four experience levels

Action

- **Research** – Videotapes of a sequence of consultations recorded during the team's normal surgeries are consensus marked by other colleagues in pairs. Feedback shows that:
    - — expert behaviour is to a significant extent dependent on case challenge. Case challenge is adapted as a case descriptor on an A to C scale, with C as the most challenging
    - — case by case, an experienced doctor will perform at competent, proficient and expert levels according to the case opportunities or challenges
    - — the meaning attributed to a *competent* consultation needs to be clarified.

> INSIGHT – Experienced doctor fingerprints range from competent to expert according to the case challenge.

> Question: How do we use the circular model to fingerprint a case more accurately and objectively?

Action

- **Discussion** – The technique of **indicative statements,** as used in the draft document *Good Medical Practice for General Practitioners* (RCGP, October 1999), is adopted as a means of identifying behaviours at different performance levels within each of the Model's domains.
- **Group** cohesion – Each project group member takes responsibility for devising indicative statements for one category. Identifying the first set of indicative statements is felt to be a significant moment in the Model's development.

> Question: Can expert consulting be identified and validated using the indicative statements?

Action

- **Research** – 'Judith Anderson', a simulation of a very complex patient case, is recorded in consultation with all eight members of the project group in their own surgeries. The resulting tapes are fingerprinted by two other members of the group and compared. Subsequently, Judith Anderson is recorded

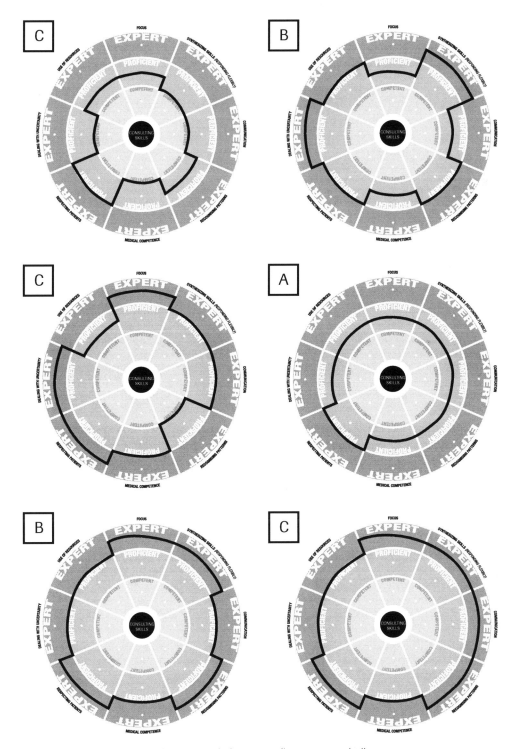

Figure A.4 Six fingerprints showing variation according to case challenge

consulting with five GPStRs and the fingerprints are compared with those of the project group.

Comparisons show that:

— all eight members of the project team's consultations extend into the expert performance level of the Model, but there is a wide range in the number of domains individual members register at expert level

— the consistency of the 'Judith Anderson' SP presentation based on a real patient according to the Leicester method is remarked upon as a reliable and uncommon research resource

— the indicative statements aid the development of appropriate fingerprints

— the comparison with GPStRs' fingerprints conform to expectations, i.e. experience is associated with increased frequency of expert behaviour.

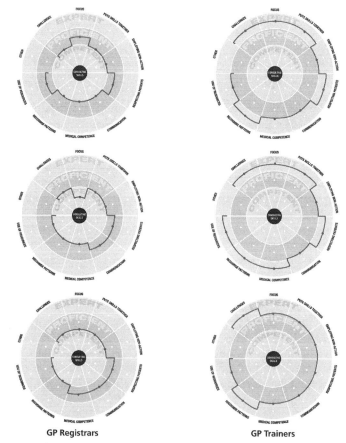

GP Registrars   **GP Trainers**

Fingerprints of consultations with the same high-challenge patient by three GP Registrars and three GP Trainers.

Figure A.5 Judith Anderson – comparison fingerprints

- **Exposure** – Three members of the group present the now four-component Model as 'work in progress' to the academic Primary Care Medical Faculty of the Catholic University, Leuven, Belgium. The Model is received with respect but with three serious reservations that prompt the next sequence of activity.

> Questions:
> ❏ How do we explain the difference between a competent, proficient and expert consultation – what is our performance typology?
> ❏ What marking key should we provide to guide colleagues making fingerprints?
> ❏ How do we propose to test the validity of the ideas incorporated in the Model and the reliability of the marking process?

Action
- **Reflection** – The three presenters in Belgium realise that all the above points would probably have been considered as intrinsic features of an academic research project. Clearly, the group is engaged in an unaccustomed practitioner style of research. Nevertheless, it is apparent the group is involved in exploring genuinely new ground.
- **Discussion** – Interest generated by the visit to Belgium results in a thorough scrutiny and rewriting of the indicative statements together with a detailed marking key (legend) for each of the categories. An attempt is made to write a descriptive typology of consulting features at each of the three performance levels. This proves to be possible for the competent and expert levels but difficult for the proficient level, which is difficult to encapsulate discretely, i.e. other than as a transition zone.
- **Specialist help engaged** – A second non-doctor member with editing and linguistic experience is invited to join the group with a brief to check the consistency and accessibility of the planned summary report. She suggests that four concepts underpin the Model. These are adopted as the four dimensions of the **Impression Graph** (Figure A.6). It soon becomes apparent that the Impression Graph can be used to improve the accuracy of the fingerprinting process by providing an impression mark to compare with the more detailed marking derived from the indicative statements – a customary methodology in educational marking. The Impression Graph also substitutes as a form of diagrammatic typology.

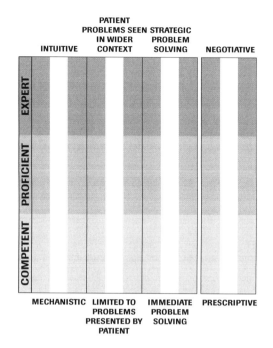

Figure A.6 Impression Graph

> INSIGHT – In an overview of the fingerprinting process, the indicative statements provide a description of the performance tree with all its leaves and minor branches. When this detail is added to an outline of the trunk and major branches provided by the Impression Graph, a more trustworthy picture emerges. Further use of the metaphor might include consulting skills as the tree's roots.

- **Consolidation** – Detailed work on the indicative statements and marking key is completed, and final aspects of the Model are shared between all members of the group.
- **Exposure** – The report *Developing GP Consulting Skills: the progression from competence to expertise* is presented to the enlarged Leicestershire, Northampton and Rutland Deanery trainers' conference (70+ members). Feedback indicates muted acceptance and some trainer interest in becoming involved with future activity.

INSIGHT – The four attributes of the Model appear to be acceptable to colleague family doctor trainers:

- ❑ consultation skills core
- ❑ eight domains
- ❑ three performance levels
- ❑ indicative statements.

It is also important to record that the development stage proceeds piecemeal, from meeting to meeting. There is no overall academic research plan and no one appears to speculate on the eventual outcome. It is an experiential journey that extends over four years.

2. Testing phase

Question: To what extent is the Model and associated fingerprinting process acceptable to colleagues outside the local family doctor trainer cohort?

Informal testing

- Exposure – The Model is presented to groups of advisers, trainers, practising family doctors and registrars. When exposing the Model at this stage, it is usual for a doctor member of the project group to explain the main features, followed by a practical fingerprinting exercise. Response sheets from experienced doctors indicate the following:

The four dimensions of the Impression Graph fit my previous experience.					
	Disagree			Agree	
	1	2	3	4	
Deanery Advisers	0	2	7	4	(13)
Lincoln Trainers	0	4	14	6	(24)
Northampton Trainers	0	1	4	7	(12)

(continued)

WONCA Europe – Amsterdam	0	2	9	2	(13)
Total feedback from 62 experienced family doctors	0	9	34	19	(62)

The eight categories of the Consultation Expertise Model provide sufficient 'fit' with my experience to encompass higher-order family doctor consulting practice

	Disagree		Agree		
	1	2	3	4	
Deanery Advisers	0	1	7	5	(13)
Lincoln Trainers	0	1	16	8	(25)
Northampton Trainers	0	0	4	8	(12)
WONCA Europe – Amsterdam	0	1	4	9	(14)
Total feedback from 62 experienced family doctors	0	3	31	30	(64)

- **Feedback** – Feedback from these sessions is affirmative, with some very specific reservations regarding the need for time to gain familiarity with the details of the Model before use. There are some specific marking difficulties: for example, discomfort with the notion of Synthesising Skills. End-of-session comments underline a positive interest in opening up the expertise dialogue. At no time does any colleague raise the issue of additional domains, or the omission of existing domains, or object to the sequence of indicative statements.

- **Presentations** are given to groups of VTS registrars in their final six months of training. On these occasions the Model is presented as a planned workshop including a specially filmed sequence of comparative consultations with the same simulated patient by a GPStR and an experienced trainer to expose experiential difference. This is followed by a fingerprinting exercise using a consultation recorded by a member of the group. The workshop is subsequently presented to groups of family doctor practitioners and family doctor trainers.

INSIGHT – The response 'The Model is too complicated' leads to deeper thinking, particularly the distinction between complicated and complex consultation approaches. It is decided that **expert consulting is complex**. Once this distinction is understood by colleagues the Model seems to become more accessible.

- **Selected feedback** from five workshop sessions with end-of-training registrars provides a picture of the reaction range:
  - *Too much information in one go – so probably won't have a great effect at the moment (Northampton VTS).*
  - *Are the criteria in each domain too vague to be applied with consistency? (Northampton VTS).*
  - *Good objective map that covers main area of consulting, is a visual tool based on complexity of the consultation and the pool of patients (Leicester VTS).*
  - *It is interesting! I particularly agree with the point that developing consulting expertise is a good way of increasing job satisfaction (Northampton VTS).*
  - *There can be various levels of expertise and all can be good. There is variation with each consultation and type of patient (Aylesbury VTS).*
  - *Good pathway, however, the self knowledge bit is missing (Aylesbury VTS).*
  - *It's a bit confusing at first as the pathway is a bit crowded but going into one bit separately was very helpful (Leicester VTS).*

INSIGHT – The experience of exposing the Model to colleagues results in an appreciation that **patient-centred consulting requires an 'intellectual leap'** in the sense that the consultant has to engage with non-linear thinking in a complex context.

Formal testing
- **Research design proposal** and **research budget** – Ethics Committee approval is needed for the kind of research design proposed. It transpires that this kind of research proposal raises issues for the Ethics Committee because of its educational nature and minimal patient connection. Financial support is received from the LNR Deanery.
- **Research approval from the Ethics Committee** – The research design is constructed to obtain a validity check on the construct of the Model and

feedback on the reliability of the fingerprinting process (*see* Appendix 2). This is to be done by recording consultations by eight trainers and eight doctors within their three years post-certification – in their own surgery – with the same simulated patient. Fingerprinting is to be completed by four experienced trainers with very basic familiarity with the Model. The results are to be analysed by an expert in examination methodology.

- **Research construct**
  - A simulation is developed from a recorded consultation with a real patient according to the Leicester method – a simulated patient named Margaret Henderson.
  - A computer programme to record the results for analysis is commissioned.
  - Doctors in both categories of experience are invited to participate in the research. Twenty doctors are recruited.
  - The patient is taken to each surgery at an agreed time. The doctor is given condensed case notes, asked to consult 'in your own way in a context where there are *no exceptional time pressures*' and told 'you may make appropriate physical examinations'. This is a first-time consultation for all the doctors.
  - Four trainers are recruited to fingerprint 16 consultation recordings. This is done over a period of two days in a conference-centre setting. Two spare consultations are used to start the marking process with a basic agreement trial. Thereafter, the marker views each of the sixteen tapes in isolation and completes a fingerprint and Impression Graph. Three members of the project team are present to observe and assist with the process.
  - The data from each Impression Graph and fingerprint is transferred to the database and sent for analysis. There are 64 sets of results.

> INSIGHT – Watching marking of the Impression Graph, it becomes clear that doctors who do not engage with the patient's lifeworld cannot securely manage the patient strategically. It is easy to observe the doctors who 'go there' in terms of entering the patient's lifeworld at various levels of engagement.

- **Research results received** – Initial reaction to the numerically presented results at one level seems to indicate a 'good enough' indication of content validity and fingerprint reliability. At another level there is a low level of agreement amongst the project group as to what the results do show. For example, the analysis shows a difference in the four markers' agreement level between different domains – there is surprisingly high agreement for Synthesising Skills and lower agreement for Use of Resources.

Over five years have passed.

'In the self-reflective spiral (of action research), the plan is prospective to action, retrospectively constructed on the basis of reflection.'[3]

Fingerprint Pack – A pack containing consent forms, fingerprinting instructions and feedback proforma is produced in a format suitable for inclusion in appraisal folders.

3. Dissemination phase

Action

- Division of work
  - — Two group members will provide feedback to the 20 doctors who have been filmed for the formal research using the Fingerprint Pack.
  - — One member will prepare a draft paper for a medical journal.
  - — Two members will advise on the preparation of a CD Rom showing how to fingerprint consultations.
  - — Three members will write a fuller account to be published in book form.
- **Context** – All the above tasks call upon new skills in technical fields involving various means to communicate the Model accessibly, bearing in mind the common response that *'it looks complicated'*.
- **CD Rom** – A 1¼ hour CD Rom is produced for colleagues' use at home or in CPD groups. Three doctors are shown on film talking through each stage of fingerprint making, based upon a recorded case they have seen previously. At the end, for practice, another doctor is recorded consulting with the same simulated patient.

> **Question:** How should the research results be presented in a medical journal paper?

'The validity of the concepts, models and results it (research) generates depends not so much on scientific tests of truth as on their utility in helping practitioners to act more effectively skilfully and intelligently.'[4]

Action

- **Paper for a professional journal** – Two problems arise:
  - — The complex nature of the Model and its research validation make condensation difficult. There is a parallel problem in choosing a presentational style suitable for an educational action research project in the medical arena. In attempting to resolve the above question, differences of opinion emerge between those who take a more quantitative and those who take a more qualitative approach. These tensions possibly reflect attitudes within the wider profession.
  - — The group as a whole continues to believe that the value of the Model lies in its practical utility. Publications were prepared by those with a relevant interest in quantitative or qualitative descriptions.
- **Publication** – A contract is signed to produce a book of no less than 120 pages. An attempt to put together a book containing contributions from all eight members of the group soon flounders on the problems of content development and style that cannot be resolved by editing. Intriguingly, in thinking through how best to portray the Model, previously unconsidered issues arise. As an unanticipated consequence, this third stage of action acquires a momentum of its own. The three authors begin to write the book incorporating other colleagues' contributions where appropriate. This proves to be difficult because of other personal and professional constraints.
- **Interpretation** – Interpretive questions arise as text for different medical audiences is considered. What, for example, do we understand by the term *consulting skills*? Expertise progression is implicit in the three performance levels and explicit in indicative statements and Impression Graph behaviours, but how do we as medical trainers propose that colleagues develop these advanced skills? The quotation below expresses what we find ourselves doing.

'The interpretive process starts with <u>describing</u> . . . The next three phases encompass the actual analysis process and include <u>organising, connecting and corroborating/legitimating</u> . . . Connecting is the operation whereby one connects various segments and emerging interpretations within the data to identify and/or discover connections, patterns, themes and new meanings.'[5]

> Question: Can we identify practical stages in the development of consulting expertise that will enable colleagues to move from competent to expert as well as affirm and provide development insights for experts?

Action

- **Fingerprinting** – Ongoing exploration of how fingerprints may be used adds to the advice bank. The conviction grows that fingerprinting can be promoted as an essential aid in charting expertise development.
- **Expertise training** – Discussion focused on interpretive use of the Impression Graph leads to a conviction that expertise can be prompted either for self-development or through formal training workshops using simulated patients by means of in-depth consideration of 'starting anywhere', which is what experts actually do; of 'going there', which represents engaging with the patient's lifeworld for therapeutic purposes; and 'concordance', which at its negotiated best symbolises both efficient and effective health gain

> INSIGHT – The columns of the Impression Graph take on added meaning when it is understood that:
> ❏ the higher level of the mechanistic-intuitive column enables expert doctors to **start anywhere**
> ❏ the middle two columns are linked by **going there**, because if the doctor does not enter the patient's lifeworld, it is not possible to deal with a case strategically
> ❏ real negotiation implies a **concordant** outcome.

> **Question:** How can we promote the Consultation Expertise Model in such a way that it will become used by colleagues?

'There are two aims of all action research: to improve and to involve. Action research aims at improvement in three areas: firstly, the improvement of a practice, secondly, the improvement of the understanding of the practice by its practitioners; and thirdly, the improvement of the situation in which the practice takes place.'[6]

Action

- **Completion** – Publication of *Advanced Consulting* leaves the above question and the axiom '*improvement of the situation in which practice takes place*' open for others to answer. It must be said, the authors have become increasingly aware of colleagues' reluctance to engage in fingerprinting without external endorsement and pressure. Possibly, time out for training may increase self-commitment. On the other hand, revalidation processes may provide external encouragement to set aside time for fingerprinting and professional reflection.

Research Process Review

On looking back, it is apparent that the quest to identify attributes of higher-order family doctor consulting, as perceived by experienced family doctor trainers at a local level, on the one hand has the benefit of being soundly practitioner-based and, on the other, has an outcome that is probably different from one conducted by professional medical researchers.

It is also apparent that the manner in which the project has progressed fits neatly into an action learning model.[7,8,9] At each stage the Model is checked with critical friends. Though unplanned, and unconscious at the time, the Model emerges stage by stage, as Kolb says, 'as a process whereby knowledge is created through the transformation of experience.'[10] In our case, it is a process extending over eight years. This may partially explain why finding a suitable medical journal format has proved to be so difficult. Essentially, action learning research of this kind fits better with an educational than with a medical research model. But educational action research is the field of small-scale practitioner activity as used by teachers, trainers and lecturers for their own local improvement projects. In our case the methodology has been applied to a problem that has very wide professional relevance. Inadvertently, we have become players in a wider pool. Potentially, the Model could help promote a major cultural shift from an acceptance of competence as the norm to one with a more developmental approach whereby the deliberate development of higher-order expertise becomes a professional expectation.

References

1. Atweh B, Kemmis S, Weeks P. *Action Research in Practice*. London: Routledge; 1998. p. 24.
2. Ibid. p. 23.
3. Carr W, Kemmis S. *Becoming Critical: education, knowledge and action research*. London: Falmer Press; 1986. p. 186.
4. Mckernan J. *Curriculum Action Research: a handbook of methods and resources for the reflective practitioner*. 2nd ed. London: Kogan Page;1996. p. 4.
5. Crabtree B, Miller W, editors. *Doing Qualitative Research*. London: Sage Publications; 1999. p. 20.
6. Carr, op cit. p. 165.
7. Ibid.
8. Atweh, Kemmis, Weeks, op cit.

9. McKernan, op cit.
10. Kolb D. *Experiential Learning: experience as the source of learning and development.* Englewood Cliffs, NJ: Prentice Hall; 1984.

THE QUESTION OF VALIDITY AND RELIABILITY

Informal testing

Generally speaking, educators do not subject new ideas to analytical scrutiny; they establish whether the idea works for them, usually by trial and error. Indeed, the Model emerged through trial and error in just that fashion. Exposure of the final Model to colleagues with various levels of experience showed that:

- the design of the Model, with the domain and performance levels radiating from a 'consulting skills' core, fits with a general understanding of family practice
- the eight consultation expertise domains resonate with practitioner experience. Furthermore, reaction has reflected a sense of completeness in that there appear to be no omissions
- at first sight, the indicative statements, as portrayed in the fully completed design, are dismissed as too complicated. With appropriate preparation, the indicative statements are found to have utility when applied to the fingerprinting of a specific case recording
- with minimal training the indicative statements are found to produce consultation fingerprints that fulfil a criterion of being 'a fair representation of what happened'.

Practitioner responses, after exposure over several years, can therefore be said to confirm **construct validity**. Given that the fingerprinting procedure is intended for formative use only, the fingerprints produced from colleague recordings are considered to be **sufficiently reliable** for the intended purpose of generating discussion and improvement.

More formal testing

It was felt necessary to subject the Model to a more exacting form of scrutiny. Ethics Committee approval was therefore obtained to conduct a small-scale enquiry according to the research design in the box below.

RESEARCH DESIGN

Twenty doctors – 10 family doctor trainers and 10 family doctors in their first three years of practice – agree to consult with the same simulated patient case and be recorded in their own consulting room.

A simulation is developed according to the Leicester method from a recording of a real patient, with appropriate patient and doctor consent.

The simulated patient (B challenge) is taken to doctors' surgeries over a period of several weeks.

Doctors are informed that they may make appropriate physical examinations (the patient has been trained) and that they should consult in their own way, in a context where there are no exceptional time pressures.

Four family doctor trainers are recruited as markers. They are given a brief marking moderation session using reserve tapes of the same case.

Markers fingerprint 16 cases alone but under supervision using four separate monitors.

The results from 64 fingerprints (including impression scores) are entered on a custom-built database and analysed by two independent examiners – one an educational examiner, the other a research statistician.

The findings are:

- Rank ordering of doctors by fingerprint and impression marks places five trainers and three new doctors in the top eight. This conflicts with the 'gold standard' assumption that all experienced trainers will consult at a higher level than newcomers, i.e. eight trainers in the top eight. This probably reflects the reality of consulting performance. It should be remembered that these scores are based on one case only.
- Marking correlation between domains reflects inter-domain relationships stated in the domain descriptions – a positive validity indicator.
- The extent of agreement between markers, an aspect of reliability, is reasonable for minimally trained markers. It is anticipated that most doctors using the method will be minimally trained.
- There is greatest marker agreement with Synthesising Skills, and least agreement with the marking of Recognising Patterns, Medical Competence and Use of Resources.

    The least agreement finding is not surprising, because:
    — Pattern Recognition can be difficult to observe, particularly if there is no

supporting information on the post-consultation Fingerprint Case Sheet

— Medical Competence requires discrete interpretation, as it refers to the application of medical knowledge and skill – it is not a test of the doctor's knowledge

— Use of Resources demands an overall judgement of at least four resources: investigation, review, referral, prescribing (time).

— Secure marking requires practice.

● Inter-assessor concordance (reliability) scores are high for all eight of the fingerprint domains and all four of the Impression Graph scales. These results are statistically significant for all domains.

● The combined fingerprint and impression scores show, as expected, that total trainer scores are higher than those for new doctors, an aspect of validity.

● Interestingly, ranking by the simulated patient produced a similar result.

Bearing in mind the small research sample, the assumption that trainers' consulting skills would be of a uniformly high standard is shown to be untrue. That notwithstanding, **the Model has been shown to be sufficiently robust for use in expertise development.**

However, even given the above endorsement, there are clearly wider questions to be asked about the nature of expert consulting. For example, do the expert-level indicative statements really encapsulate the higher levels of expertise? How achievable are these or similar high levels in today's primary care culture? More apposite perhaps for the project group, will the fingerprinting process prove to be useful in encouraging doctors to aspire to more advanced consulting behaviour? These and other questions remain for others to pursue.

As Patricia Benner says of the Dreyfus model of skill acquisition:

> *'This is a situational model of skill acquisition, as opposed to a trait or talent model. Since this model is situational, performance level can be determined only by consensual validation of expert judges (other doctors!) and assessment of the outcomes of a situation. Reliability is determined by inter-rater agreement between experts by repeated assessment.'*[1]

Ultimately, as this is not an assessment model, colleagues will make their own validity and reliability decisions as they use or don't use the Consultation Expertise Model.

One final thought: does the fact that we have been able to echo the thoughts of many medical writers with quotations in the text provide another modicum of validity?

Reference

1. Benner P. *From Novice to Expert: excellence and power in clinical nursing practice.* New Jersey: Prentice Hall; 1984. p. 293.

APPENDIX 3   THE USE OF SIMULATED PATIENTS

THE DISTINCTIVE LEICESTER SIMULATED-PATIENT METHOD

The brand of simulated patient we have taken so much for granted is distinctive to our Leicester locality and is as much the result of local initiative as the Consultation Expertise Model itself.

Simulated patients developed according to the Leicester model are firmly based on real patients who have formally consented to doctors recording their consultation on film. This enables the simulator not only to adopt the symptoms but also to adapt to the demeanour, tone of voice and physical movements and, in conversation with the originating doctor, to become aware of the social circumstances of the actual patient. While the simulator cannot replicate the original patient, s/he can, matched for age and gender, *represent* the patient. After several trial consultations, accompanied by anonymised clinical notes derived from the real patient, the simulator can present a near-reality patient experience.

> Simulated patients: the Leicester method
> ❏   Doctor films consultations with consent.
> ❏   Simulator chooses a patient s/he feels able to bond with.
> ❏   Simulator studies recording for verbal and non-verbal behaviour.
> ❏   Doctor and simulator meet to discuss symptoms and known social background of original patient.
> ❏   Simulator tries role with originating doctor.
> ❏   Doctor prepares case notes.
> ❏   Simulator consults with other doctors to explore and test out the role. The role is given a name.

It's the identification with a real patient that makes this approach distinctive. With the original recording in mind, when doctors ask unexpected questions simulators can ask themselves, 'What would the original patient have said or done?' By comparison, scenario-based simulations, though frequently based on real patient experiences, are devised by doctors and learned from a written description by simulators. The character of the patient has thus to be grafted on by the simulator.

As mentioned above, simulators can only represent, not replicate the original patient, so simulators have to respond in a manner consistent with the original patient when something new comes up. Let's say an out-of-the-blue question such as 'Do you have dogs at home?' It is understood practice that whatever answer is given becomes integrated into the role forever. This has been given the label *creative consistency*.

All simulators have to avoid colluding with doctors by not feeding answers, i.e. maintaining the integrity of being a patient. Similarly they have to acquire the habit of cleansing themselves of previous consultations so they can respond naturally to each new doctor. For a fuller description of the Leicester method, see Thew and Worrall.[1]

SIMULATED PATIENTS: AN INTEGRAL FACTOR IN THE DEVELOPMENT OF THE CONSULTATION EXPERTISE MODEL

Simulated patients were used on three occasions to help explore aspects of the Model's development. Each of these activities has led to further learning.

1. Simulated patients were used to test the notion that expertise is dependent on length of experience

This was tested practically by filming 10-minute consultations with three simulated patients by:

- two year-four medical students
- two family doctor specialty training registrars
- two newly qualified family doctors
- two experienced family doctors.

The patient presentations were based on patients recorded by members of the development group chosen to provide a representation of typical day-to-day patients.

- Susan Maughan – a 48-year-old mother of two children with a history of depression who presents for a repeat prescription and to report how well she now feels. She is worried about the constipation side effects and the extent to which the antidepressants affect her HRT implant and the timing of its renewal.
- Mike Bellamy – a 35-year-old motor mechanic has a continuing pain in the ribs where he fell over (he'd been to casualty), he feels ill, 'fluey' and sweaty and has not been to work for a week. He also wants to talk about the effects of drinking and smoking on his life.

- Cathy Wilkes – a 41-year-old asthmatic has a bad cough and asks for antibiotics. She has been taking her thyroid tablets irregularly, is casual about using her inhalers and is desperate to stay well enough to work.

All the consultations take place on the same evening in a health centre in standard family doctor consulting rooms observed only by the camera. Bearing in mind that the volunteer medical students and young doctors were invited to take part in this trial because of their known worth, scrutiny of the 24 recordings suggested that the basic hypothesis of expertise being dependent on experience appeared to be the case. This is only possible because patient simulators can wipe previous consultations from their minds and present as first-time patients to each of the eight consultants.

2. Simulated patients were used to explore expert consulting in more detail

In order to explore expert behaviour in detail it was decided to use each project group member as a guinea pig and film them consulting with an acknowledged complex, challenging patient in their own consulting room. For this a simulation was developed based on a patient seen by a colleague outside the group. The simulated patient taken to eight surgeries was:

- Judith Anderson – a 63-year-old married woman with a 40-year history of depression, varied medication and symptoms akin to Parkinson's disease for which she is being seen by the neurologist who has not so far identified the cause. She presents holding a Nexium packet in her shaking hand but can't remember why she has come. She remembers later that she wants to reduce the dose. She asks if she can have a brain scan and describes being confused and losing her sense of balance.

The recordings were fingerprinted by two of the development group, whose objectivity was put to the test when fingerprinting. They used the then newly adopted indicative statements. The simulator also completed post-consultation reflection sheets. The idiosyncratic nature of each of the eight consultations illustrates just how – because the simulator becomes the patient – she can react credibly to different doctor approaches and, as a consequence, enable comparisons to be made for research purposes.

3. Simulated patients were used to test the validity and reliability of the Model

Not unnaturally, a simulated patient was used when it came to formal research design. In order to test the validity of the Model and the reliability of the fingerprinting process, a simulation was developed to provide a standard of comparison between 20 doctors again filmed in their own consulting rooms.

- Margaret Henderson – a 49-year-old married woman under specialist care for COPD, on HRT following a hysterectomy 10 years ago, who presents with recurrent backache.

This patient was taken to 20 different surgeries and the resulting recordings were fingerprinted by four experienced family doctor trainers. Despite the individuality of each doctor's consultation, the credibility of the patient was never called into question, so an uninterrupted focus on the behaviour of the doctor was possible. An example of how this can occur in detail can be seen in the analysis of three transcripts of the Margaret Henderson case as used previously to illustrate fingerprinting.

It is possible the search for a means to identify the nature of expert consulting would not have progressed beyond local interest were it not for the easy availability of validated 'standardised' simulated patients. Validated in the sense that patients prepared according to the Leicester method have previously been accredited by research for their use in the assessment of consulting competence for family doctor certification – summative assessment by simulated patient surgery, whereby candidates see eight patients assessed at a high pass level and a further eight if they do not pass through that screen.[2] The consistency of these simulated patient presentations has thus been found acceptable nationally for high-stake assessment. For research purposes it only remains necessary to quality check each new simulation, a process aided by the use of very experienced simulators.

References

1. Thew R, Worrall P. The selection and training of patient simulators for the assessment of consultation performance in simulated surgeries. *Educ Gen Pract.* 1998; 9(2): 211–15.
2. Allen J, Evans A, Foulkes J, *et al.* Simulated surgery in the assessment of general practice training: results of a trial in the Trent and Yorkshire region. *Br J Gen Pract.* 1998; **48**: 1219–23.

APPENDIX 4 FINGERPRINT PACK

The contents of this pack can be downloaded from the following web address: http://www.eastmidlandsdeanery.nhs.uk/document_store/12253605961_fingerprint_pack.pdf

Developing GP Consulting Skills:

the progression from competence to expertise

CONSULTATION EXPERTISE MODEL

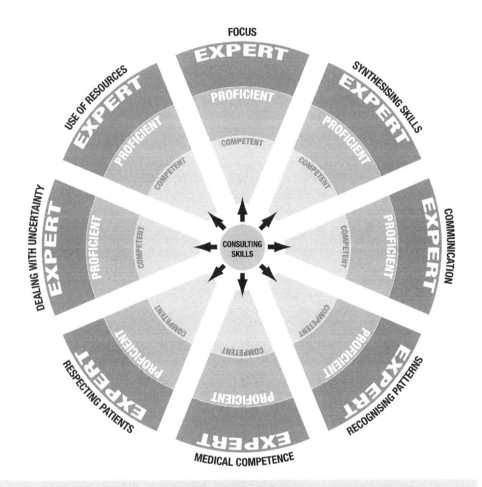

FINGERPRINT PACK

Developing GP Consulting Skills:

the progression from competence to expertise | **CONSULTATION EXPERTISE MODEL**

Using the Consultation Expertise Model

The model has been developed in order to:

- Help doctors develop expertise through reflective practice.
- Provide evidence of expertise for appraisal and revalidation.

Most well-known consultation models aim to demonstrate that a doctor can function at more than a basic level of competence for the purposes of certification. This model provides an opportunity to demonstrate progression towards and possession of higher levels of competence and expertise. Basic or minimal competence should be demonstrated in other ways. Usually the model will be used by confident consulters. Such confidence usually requires wide ranging consulting experience.

Because the model has been designed to identify expertise, it is recommended that, when using it to look at a consultation, colleagues should seek to identify behaviour that is expert or nearly so by using the indicative statements.

During the feedback dialogue there is an opportunity to highlight existing expert behaviour and to identify situations where, with practice, expertise can be attained.

Not all expert doctors will demonstrate expert behaviours in all consultations. This may be because the issues presented do not require expert behaviour. However, over a number of consultations, an expert doctor can demonstrate expert behaviours in each of the categories of the model.

Developing GP Consulting Skills:

the progression from competence to expertise   **FINGERPRINTING CHECKLIST**

ENCLOSED PAPERWORK
- Patient Consent Form
- Conditions Governing Tapes
- Fingerprint Case Sheet
- Impression Graph Sheet
- Fingerprint Sheet
- CATEGORIES - indicative statements
- Six case Fingerprint Sheet
- Six case Impression Graph
- Feedback Guidance
- Feedback Sheets 1 & 2
- Reflection Sheet

Stage 1

☐ Record patient consultation(s) with consent(s).
Check tape compatibility - VHS/digital?

☐ Complete Fingerprint Case Sheet – the cover for each consultation.

☐ Confirm conditions governing recordings and arrange exchange of recorded
consultation(s) with colleague familiar with LNR Trainers' Model.

EITHER

(a) Agree to view recordings privately, complete fingerprint and arrange
feedback meeting.

Or

(b) As colleagues, decide to view and rate each others tapes together, engaging
in feedback dialogue as each consultation is reviewed.

Stage 2
Fingerprinting a Consultation

☐ View consultation using Feedback Sheets to record observations.

☐ Rate (review) consultation on *Impression Graph*.

☐ Use *indicative statements* in all eight categories to produce a case fingerprint
(use NA = not applicable, if it's not appropriate to mark a category)

- be guided by the *indicative statements* - 'did you see this happen?'
- record observation and comments on *Feedback Sheet*.
- mark each category to the selected point, i.e. to one of the seven dots.
- when all eight categories are marked review case challenge judgement, then record your A-B-C judgement on right side of *Fingerprint Case Sheet*.
- compare performance level of categories fingerprint with the impression marking.

☐ Decide on issues for feedback, remembering specifically to include areas requested from the consulter for feedback.

Stage 3
Hold Feedback Discussion

- confirm what specific feedback colleague wants in relation to expertise.
- provide feedback according to LNR Trainers' Model feedback guidance.
- hold open discussion.
- record learning or practice needs on learning plan.

Stage 4
Reflect on Practice

- write reflective summary to complete *Reflection Sheet* and include with supporting fingerprint evidence in appraisal portfolio envelope.

Developing GP Consulting Skills:

the progression from competence to expertise | **PATIENT INFORMATION SHEET**

Please take time to read this sheet. If you are unclear ask the receptionist or doctor.

Your doctor is recording some consultations today as part of normal medical training processes. You will be asked to sign a form consenting to this.

What will happen if I agree to my consultation being videotaped?

The videotape of your consultation will be seen by your doctor and another GP doctor. No one else will see the tape. The doctors will analyse what happens on the tape so that your doctor can plan future education and learning.

What happens to the tape after it has been seen?

After both doctors have seen the tape it will be destroyed.
It is your own doctor's responsibility to do this.

What happens if I don't want my examination to be recorded?

Tell the doctor who will pause the tape until you are happy to continue the recording.
(No intimate examination is ever videotaped).

What will happen if I change my mind about being videotaped?

Tell your doctor who will wipe or destroy the tape immediately.

What will happen if I don't want to be videotaped?

That is perfectly OK. Tell the receptionist or the doctor and the video machine will be switched off.
Your clinical care will not be affected if you do not wish to be videotaped.

Please note

■ **Video recordings are carried out according to National Training Guidelines.**
■ **Videotapes are subject to the same degree of confidentiality as all other medical records.**

PATIENT CONSENT FORM

Please initial box

I confirm that I have read and understand the information sheet and have the opportunity to ask questions.

☐

I understand that my participation is voluntary and I am free to withdraw at any time, without giving reason, without my medical care or legal rights being affected.

☐

I agree to my consultation being videotaped.

☐

Before

_____ _____ _____

Name of patient   Date   Signature

_____ _____ _____

Name of person taking consent   Date   Signature

After

_____ _____ _____

Patient   Date   Signature

_____ _____ _____

Doctor   Date   Signature

Developing GP Consulting Skills:

the progression from competence to expertise | **CONDITIONS GOVERNING TAPES**

Conditions governing the presentation of patient consultation videotapes for fingerprinting

- Fingerprints of patient consultations using the Consultation Expertise Model are intended for reflection on professional practice.

- It is anticipated that fingerprints will be used for personal feedback, peer discussion, or appraisal evidence as determined by the consulting doctor.

- The tapes will only be seen either, by a doctor familiar with the Consultation Expertise Model fingerprinting procedure or, by colleagues using the Fingerprinting Pack.

- Both patients and doctors are entitled to have their confidentiality protected. Confidentiality will therefore be maintained by all concerned *subject to normal governance procedures*.

- Fully completed patient consent forms for each consultation should be kept by the consulting doctor.

- It is recommended that a maximum of six consultations should be considered.

- A Fingerprint Case Sheet should accompany each consultation to provide fingerprinters with relevant information not apparent on the recording.

- Tapes should be of good visual and sound quality with a clear view of the doctor and the patient's body language. Fingerprinting doctors are entitled to omit recordings of poor quality.

- It is anticipated that feedback will be provided in the form of a fingerprint and case challenge grading and that reference to the indicative statements in the eight categories of the model and impression graph will provide opportunity for personal reflection. Alternatively, peer feedback may be arranged according to pre-determined criteria.

- Feedback will be on a non-judgemental, no fault basis. Should differences of opinion arise it is important that they are treated at the level of professional dialogue the model is designed to foster.

- Fingerprint information belongs to the consulting doctor.

Signed Dr ....Consulting Doctor   Date ....

Signed Dr ....Fingerprinter   Date ....

Developing GP Consulting Skills:
the progression from competence to expertise | **FINGERPRINT CASE SHEET**

NOTES of CASE	Patient Age

Reasons for attendance

Patients' previous events

Doctor's previous contact

What affected you most in the consultation (thoughts and feelings)

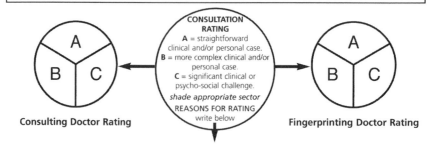

Consulting Doctor Rating

CONSULTATION
RATING
A = straightforward clinical and/or personal case.
B = more complex clinical and/or personal case.
C = significant clinical or psycho-social challenge.
shade appropriate sector
REASONS FOR RATING
write below

Fingerprinting Doctor Rating

Developing GP Consulting Skills:

the progression from competence to expertise | **IMPRESSION GRAPH**

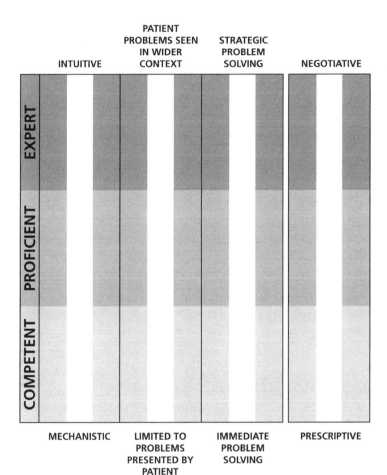

How to use the Impression Graph
- Use the graph to register an **impression** of the consultation performance position on each of the four dimensions.
- After completing impression levels on each of the four dimensions, draw a judgment line to establish a performance level for the consultation. This overall impression can then be used as a point of reference when engaged in the detail of fingerprinting.

Forming an Impression: some points to consider
- Pay attention to 'fluency' - does it look easy? Experts are renowned for making a task look easy.
- Get a sense of how reactive-proactive the doctor is to the patient - this has influence on all four dimensions.
- Information on the Fingerprint Sheet may be particularly helpful for the intuitive-mechanistic dimension as it might be possible to gain an insight into the doctor's inner thoughts.
- Impression marks on the negotiation-prescription dimension should be patient related - negotiation may be inappropriate in some cases.

Developing GP Consulting Skills:

the progression from competence to expertise | SIX IMPRESSION GRAPH SHEET

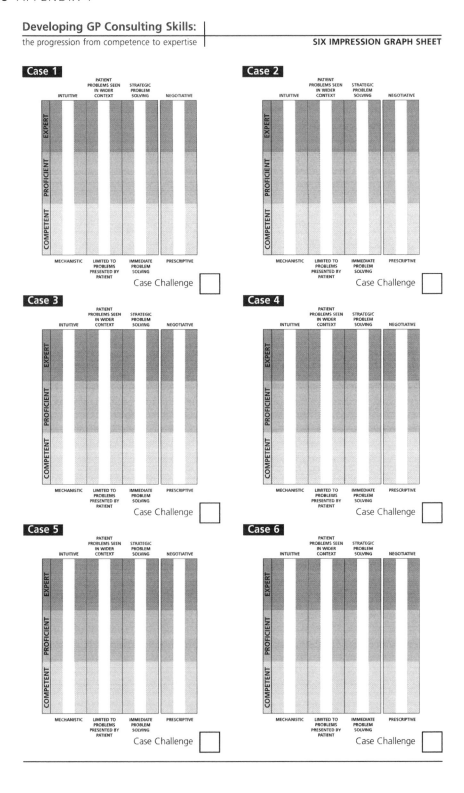

Developing GP Consulting Skills:
the progression from competence to expertise | **FINGERPRINT SHEET**

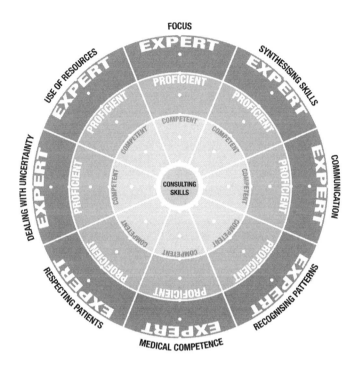

Marking Sheet

Case	Case Challenge

Drawing Fingerprints

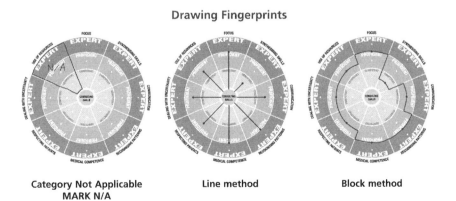

Category Not Applicable   Line method   Block method
MARK N/A

Developing GP Consulting Skills:
the progression from competence to expertise

SIX CONSULTATION FINGERPRINT

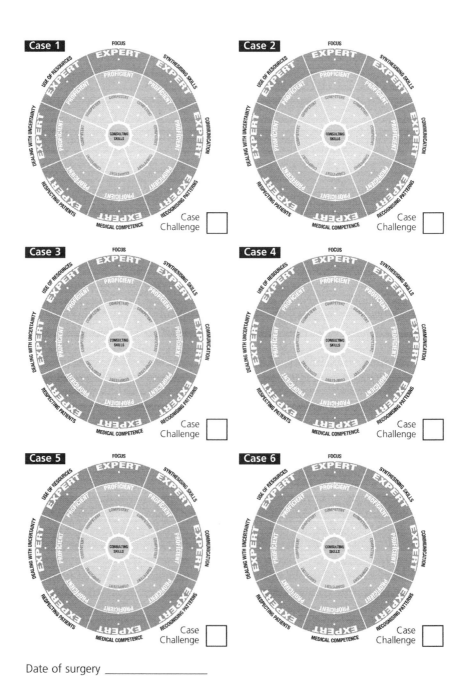

Date of surgery _____

The Feedback and Reflection Sheets

The *Feedback and Reflection Sheets* provide a basic feedback structure to assist colleagues sustain and develop consulting expertise. They should not in any way restrict a robust professional dialogue or record of whatever is felt to be useful. Bearing that in mind, it is worth noting some constraints on feedback exchange that have become apparent from previous experience.

■ GPs unaccustomed to giving face-to-face consultation analysis are often overly sensitive to colleague feelings.

■ There may initially be a tendency to overestimate the level of a colleague's consultation because of the above.

■ A less than frank exchange does nobody any favours. The purpose of feedback is to affirm and question observed behaviours in order to prompt attention to expertise development. Consulting doctors have a right of reply in the Reflection Sheet. Remember, it helps the consulting doctor to have statements upon which to reflect.

■ New doctors rarely have sufficient experience to be expert and should be prepared for more modest results.

■ Experienced colleagues may have slipped into habits that need challenging.

Feedback Guidelines

■ Avoid value judgements of the good - bad variety.

■ Start feedback with neutral statements based on observed behaviours. Sound advice is always to use active verbs, (when the patient said…, I heard you say… etc).

■ Stick to specifics, what you saw and heard, not what you think the patient might have meant.

■ Use the impression graph, fingerprint and observed behaviour notes to determine initial written and verbal comments.

■ Most experienced doctors have outlived Pendleton rules - always elicit what feedback your colleague wants, and how strong a level of challenge is welcome.

Using Fingerprint Feedback for Appraisal and Revalidation Portfolios

The LNR fingerprinting promotes:

• Judgements about the challenge level of the videotaped consultation by the colleague viewing the case. This is often a determining factor in the level of expertise demanded.

• Specific judgements made on the *Impression Graph* to prompt discussion on the four dimensions underpinning the model.

• The opportunity to give detailed feedback based on the indicative statements within each of the eight categories of expertise. Such detailed identification of consulting behaviour provides a second prompt for developmental discussion.

• The opportunity to reflect on the feedback and consider how it might affect future practice. This stage is essential if the fingerprinting process is to be used as evidence for appraisal, outcomes should be captured on the learning plan.

Developing GP Consulting Skills:

the progression from competence to expertise | FEEDBACK SHEET 1

Case	Feedback Date

FEEDBACK - KEY POINTS

Feedback should be based on observed behaviours, what might have been done differently and specific request by the doctor concerned.

IMPRESSION GRAPH - KEY POINTS

OBSERVED BEHAVIOURS	COMMENTS
Mechanistic - Intuitive	
Problems presented by patient - Problems seen in wider context	
Immediate problem solving - Strategic problem solving	
Prescription - Negotiation	

FINGERPRINT - KEY POINTS

OBSERVED BEHAVIOURS	COMMENTS
Communication	
Recognising Patterns	
Medical Competence	

Developing GP Consulting Skills:

the progression from competence to expertise   **FEEDBACK SHEET 2**

FINGERPRINT - KEY POINTS (CONTINUED)

OBSERVED BEHAVIOURS	COMMENTS
Respecting Patients	
Dealing with Uncertainty	
Use of Resources	
Focus	
Synthesising Skills	

FINGERPRINT CASE SHEET - KEY POINTS

Thoughts about case challenge

OVERALL IMPRESSION

Feedback Doctor signature_____

Developing GP Consulting Skills:

the progression from competence to expertise

Case(s)	Date completed

FEEDBACK POINTS REFLECTIONS
(to be completed by consulting doctor)

What needs to be included in the learning plan?

INDEX

10-year rule 165

agenda-led approach (ALOBA) 113
appraisal and revalidation 3, 9, 129, 132–3, 155, 187
attendance 123

behaviour change, in doctors 160
biases 144–5

clinical problem framing and solving skills 24–5, 30
  case example 25–6
communication skills
  case examples 35–6, 73–4
  example of feedback 120
  improving 154–5
  and interpersonal skills 146
  markings 75
  simulated case example 35
completeness 25, 47, 96–7
concordance 15, 27, 33, 46, 120, 155–6, 158–61, 168–9, 189
conscious naivety 1
consent forms 69, 106–7, 133–4, 138
consultation 36, 105
  assumptions in 38
  mapping 2–3; *see also* fingerprints
  models of 9, 31, 156, 171
  other influences on 29
  role of doctor in 30
Consultation Expertise Model 2, 14–15, 138
  appraisal and revalidation 132–3
  assumptions of 9, 11, 13, 20, 106–7, 168
  complexity of 14, 131–2, 185

  components of 17–19, 130
  concordance in 161
  context 5–6
  development of 174–90, 197
  for doctor trainers 142
  doctor's experience of 133–40
  in expertise teaching programme 170–1
  feedback in 110, 113
  feedback on process 141–2
  group use 140–1
  growth of consulting skills 31
  guidance in 168
  importance of performance levels in 102
  introducing to colleagues 129–31, 135–6
  key concepts 144
  learning concepts 168
  limits of 15
  marking problems 110, 112
  next-stage suggestions 3
  objectivity of 8, 135
  and patient lifeworld 154
  performance levels in 66
  place of impression graph 103
  postgraduate training 140
  providing a new language 5
  purpose of 2, 6, 101–2, 129, 170
  reasons for development of 60
  self-reflection 138
  summary of advanced consulting 96–7
  in teaching programmes 171–2
  validity and reliability 192–5, 198
  value of 7–9, 14, 31
  visual components of 101
  who it can be used by 7
Consultation Observation Tool (COT) 133

consulting skills 17, 20–2, 31–2
case example 32–3
components of 21
person of doctor and 31
Continuing Professional Development (CPD) 3, 6
core skills 31

dealing with uncertainty 45–7, 159
case examples 46–9, 84, 86–7
example of 159
example of feedback 122
fingerprint markings 85, 87
in making of fingerprint 109
direction of travel 163, 167
doctor–patient relationship 47, 56–8, 107, 112, 131–2
domains of expertise 18
Dreyfus model of skill acquisition 61–3, 66, 103, 146, 194
Dreyfus typology 103–4

emotions
conveyed non-verbally 34
of doctor 33
ethical dilemmas 40
experienced doctors
how they act 66–7
how they work 23
what they do 1–2, 6, 23, 27, 36, 111
evidence-based medicine (EBM) 24, 40, 58, 159
expertise, defined 102
expertise concepts 161, 172

feedback 113
from colleagues 165
doctor's reflections on 127
Feedback Sheet 108
general recommendations for 113–14, 116
indicative statements as 168
interpersonal skill observations 20
issues for 109
on Model process 141
need for 8, 113
from patients 15
process models 113

simulated case example 116–27
starting points for 112
use of fingerprints in 106, 110, 114, 120–5
use of impression graph in 115, 120
Feedback Pack 115
Fingerprint Pack 3, 101, 107–8, 110, 129, 134, 138, 200
fingerprints
analysis 67
Case Sheet 107–9, 114, 135–6, 138
development of concept 189
doctor's reflections on 127
graphic example 124
and impression graph 104–5
introduction to 2–3, 101
introductory exercise 129–30
making 107–9
multiple-case 110
observed consultation 109–10
process 3, 6–7
purpose of 105–6
reliability of 186
use of for feedback 106, 110, 114, 120–7
fluency 63, 96, 104, 112, 115, 150
focus 53–4
case examples 54–6, 90, 92–3
example of 160
example of feedback about 122
fingerprint markings 91, 93
in making of fingerprint 109

generative effect 58
'going there' 40, 47, 54, 74, 93, 115, 155–8, 168–9, 189

heuristics 47, 97, 144, 151
history building 153

impression graph 101–2, 108, 135
approaches to marking 104–5
best fit line 105, 112
and clusters of skills 170
development of 102, 181–3, 186, 189
doctor's experience of 135–6
and fingerprinting 104, 108–9
graphic example 124
and higher-level expertise 168

and intuition 151–2
and patient lifeworld 154
and performance levels 169
purposes of 103
themes of 102–3
use of in feedback 115, 120
indicative statements
defined 19, 65
case examples 67, 70
developing specific behaviours 109
doctor's experience of 135
at expert level 168
as guidance 142
limitations of 110
in making a fingerprint 108
simulated case examples 70
use of 66–7, 103, 108, 112, 138–9
interpersonal skills
case example 28–9
extended 34, 147–9
feedback 20
interpersonal skill language 146
making fingerprint 108
intuition 37–8, 64, 103, 112, 150–2
synonymous with know-how 64

know-how 12, 63–4, 172; see also intuition

learning organisations 165–6
learning support 165
Leicester Assessment Package (LAP) 5, 175
life experience 28
lifeworld of patient 11, 25, 103, 155–6, 167,
    186

management plan 28
medical competence 40–1, 112
case examples 41, 46, 78, 80
feedback 121
fingerprint markings 79
in making of fingerprint 109
medical knowledge and skill 23, 30, 40
case example 23–4
metacognition 12–13
Miller Triangle 12–13
mind map 10
mindlines 151

mindset 163–4
Model, the, see Consultation Expertise Model

negotiation 33, 46, 120, 141, 148–9, 189

patient-centred approach
accomodation in real practice 155, 166
as basis of Model 7, 11
conflicting with EBM 159
not widespread in professional practice 131
patients
individuality of 42
values and beliefs of 40
pattern recognition, see recognising patterns
performance levels 18–19, 31
defined 60
assessment 66
based on Dreyfus model 65
in nMRCGP 66
tracking 169
typology of 102
personal development plan (PDP) 115, 170
phenomenology 153
PowerPoint presentations 130
practitioners with special interests (PwSI)
    166
presence 55
case examples 55
problem framing 24–5, 32, 50, 144–5; see also
    clinical problem framing and solving skills

recognising patterns
as bias 144
case examples 37–9, 75, 77
example of 157
example of feedback 121
fingerprint markings 76–7
and intuition 150–1
making fingerprint 108
reflection sheet 136–7
respecting patients 42–4, 89, 112
case examples 44–5, 81, 83
example of 157, 160
example of feedback 121
fingerprint markings 82, 84
in making of fingerprint 109
revalidation, see appraisal and revalidation

risk analysis 46
rules of thumb, *see* heuristics

self-awareness, doctor's 112
self-blaming 84
shared decision making 16, 25, 34, 131–2,
    161
short-cuts 144, 151; *see also* heuristics
simulations 2, 5–6
    case examples 34, 67–71, 73–5, 77–8, 80–1,
        83–4, 86–7, 89–90, 92–3, 95–6
    Leicester method 196–9
    protocols of 69
    in teaching programmes 171
situational awareness 54
skills
    acquisition 8, 113, 194
    core 31
    tacit 74
'starting anywhere' 156, 168–9, 189
strategic thinking 103, 105
summative assessment 6, 14, 106
synthesising skills 40, 56–9, 112
    case examples 59, 93, 95–6

development of concept 184, 187
example of 157, 159
example of feedback about 122
expert level descriptor 124
fingerprint markings 94–5
in making of fingerprint 109
necessity for 58

tacit behaviour 11–12, 31
tacit knowledge 23, 61, 152
teaching programmes 170–2
thin slicing 38, 151

uncertainty 47–8
use of resources 49–51
    case examples 50–2, 87, 89
    development of concept 187
    example of feedback 122
    fingerprint markings 88, 90
    in making of fingerprint 109

value judgements 2

websites 153